COMMUNITY-ACQUIRED PNEUMONIA

A Plan for Implementing National Guidelines at the Local Hospital Level

Julio A. Ramirez, MD, FACP

COMMUNITY-ACQUIRED PNEUMONIA

A Plan for Implementing National Guidelines at the Local Hospital Level

Julio A. Ramirez, MD, FACP

Professor of Medicine
Chief, Division of Infectious Diseases
University of Louisville School of Medicine
Chief, Infectious Diseases
Department of Veterans Affairs Medical Center
Louisville, Kentucky

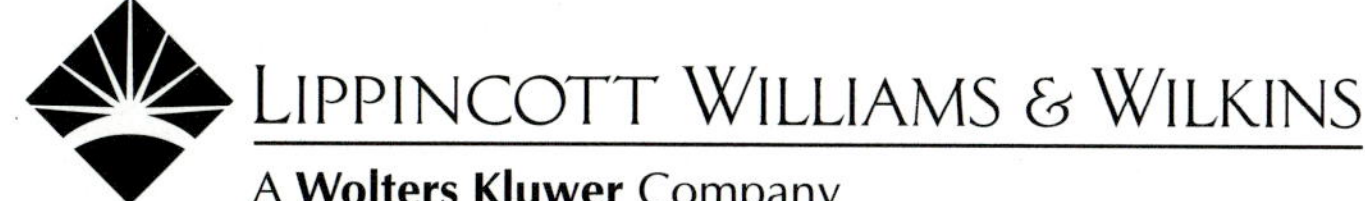

Philadelphia • Baltimore • New York • London
Buenos Aires • Hong Kong • Sydney • Tokyo

Editor: Hal Pollard
Managing Editor: Jennifer Kullgren
Marketing Manger: Julie Sikora
Purchasing Manager, Clinical and Healthcare: *Jennifer Jett*
Compositor: Maryland Composition
Printer: Walsworth Publishing

530 Walnut Street
Philadelphia, PA 19106 USA
LWW.com

Printed in the USA

Library of Congress Cataloging-in-Publication Data
(US Copyright Registration Number: Txu1-019-198)

Ramirez, Julio A., M.D.
Commmunity-acquired pneumonia : a plan for implementing national guidelines at the local hospital level / Julio A. Ramirez.
p. ; cm.
Includes bibliograpical references and index.
ISBN 0-7817-4483-0
1. Pneumonia—Patients—Hospital care—Standards. 2. Medical protocols.
[DNLM: 1. Pneumonia—therapy. 2. Community-Acquired Infections—therapy. 3. Guideline Adherence. 4. Hospitals, Community. 5. Practice Guidelines. WC 202 R173c 2003] I. Title.
RA644.P8 R365 2003
616.2′4106—dc21
2002015770

---

01 02 03 04
1 2 3 4 5 6 7 8 9 10

Table of Contents

Preface vii

Acknowledgments ix

Chapter 1: Process for Implementing a Local Practice Guideline 1

Chapter 2: Clinical Diagnosis of Pneumonia 8

Chapter 3: Need for Hospitalization 13

Chapter 4: Respiratory Isolation 17

Chapter 5: Microbiologic Workup 21

Chapter 6: Empiric Antimicrobial Therapy 24

Chapter 7: Switch from Intravenous to Oral Therapy 30

Chapter 8: Hospital Discharge 35

Chapter 9: Patient Education and Satisfaction with Care 40

Chapter 10: Clinical Outcome 43

Chapter 11: Prevention of Pneumonia 49

Appendix 52

Index 65

Preface

During the last decade, different medical and governmental organizations developed practice guidelines for the management of hospitalized patients with community-acquired pneumonia (CAP). These documents describe what can be defined as the "recommended care" of hospitalized patients with CAP based on the current scientific evidence. The ultimate goal of national guidelines is to move the local actual practice closer to the ideal practice recommended by these guidelines. In an attempt to reach this goal, national guideline documents were disseminated to institutions and health care personnel involved in the management of patients with CAP. It was supposed that such dissemination of national guidelines would alter care at the local level. At the present time, however, it is clear that relying on the passive dissemination of practice guidelines as the sole methodology to influence a change in practice is doomed to failure.

To drive local practice closer to the practice recommended by national guidelines, it is necessary to have an appropriate implementation plan. Why are the majority of institutions not implementing guidelines at the local level? One of the primary reasons is that health care workers in general are not aware of the process for guideline implementation.

The intent of this book is to outline a plan for implementation of a CAP practice guideline at the local hospital level. The recommendations described herein are based on a review of the literature in the area of practice guidelines as well as the author's personal experience in developing and implementing CAP practice guidelines at the University of Louisville–affiliated hospitals.

As health systems struggle to improve quality of care with limited resources, the pressures to develop and implement CAP practice guidelines more effectively are bound to grow. This book is intended to help physicians, pharmacists, nurses, hospital administrators, and other health care workers interested in the implementation of national guidelines for the management of patients with CAP at the local hospital level.

Acknowledgments

This publication would not have been possible without the contributions of members of the Division of Infectious Diseases of the University of Louisville. Multiple ideas suggested by different members of our clinical research group have been incorporated into this book. I also would like to thank Ginny Sciortino for her invaluable assistance in the preparation of the manuscript. Finally, I would like to thank my mentors for their guidance and my family for their continuous support.

1

Process for Implementing a Local Practice Guideline

The Need for Local Implementation
Step 1: Defining Local Quality Indicators
The Hospital Pneumonia Team • Areas of Practice with High Impact on Outcome • Local Recommended Care • Quality Indicators
Step 2: Collection and Evaluation of Data on Quality Indicators
Actual Care • Evaluation of Variance
Step 3: Interventions for Improvement
Unjustified Variance • Changing Health Care Practice
Step 4: Recollection and Evaluation of Data on Quality Indicators
Summary
References

THE NEED FOR LOCAL IMPLEMENTATION

The first US national guidelines for the management of patients with community-acquired pneumonia (CAP) were published by the American Thoracic Society (ATS) in 1993.[1] Since then, some other national organizations have published documents that deal with several aspects of the management of CAP. These organizations include the Infectious Diseases Society of America (IDSA),[2] the Centers for Disease Control and Prevention (CDC),[3] and the American College of Emergency Physicians.[4] Revised guidelines from the ATS have recently been published.[5]

The primary goals of all governmental and medical specialty organizations that develop national guidelines for the management of CAP are to improve patient outcome and/or decrease cost of care. One of the elements critical to achieving these goals is that national guidelines need to alter physician practice patterns. The initial premise was that dissemination of national guidelines would alter care at the local level. Although a tremendous amount of resources are being expended in the development and dissemination of national guidelines, there is very little evidence that the plethora of recommendations has significantly influenced medical practice. The strategy of passive dissemination of national guidelines at the local hospital level as the sole methodology to influence a change in practice proved to be unsuccessful. Today, it is clear that to move local practice closer to the practice recommended by national guidelines, it is necessary to have an appropriate plan for local implementation.

The plan for local implementation of national guidelines for hospitalized patients with CAP described in this chapter can be summarized in the following four steps: (1) development of quality indicators, (2) collection of data on quality indicators, (3) formulation of interventions for improvement, and (4) recollection of data on quality indicators.

STEP 1: DEFINING LOCAL QUALITY INDICATORS

The Hospital Pneumonia Team

A multidisciplinary team of health care workers should be formed and given the responsibility to develop and implement the hospital CAP practice guideline. This hospital "pneumonia team" is usually composed of physicians with experience in the management of patients with CAP, as well as representatives from pharmacy, nursing, microbiology, emergency medicine, respiratory therapy, radiology, hospital administration, and any other group participating in some aspect of the care of hospitalized patients with CAP. It is important for the team to be supported by a strong administrative mandate.

The first task of the pneumonia team is to create a brief document with the local recommendations for the care of hospitalized patients with CAP. National guideline documents offer a systematic review of the CAP literature and can be used as a template to develop the local document, but it is important to avoid some of the drawbacks of national guidelines. Members of national committees are primarily pulmonary and infectious diseases specialists with experience in clinical research in the area of CAP. These groups of experts will produce documents characterized by a very comprehensive review of the literature in the area of CAP. Because this approach is necessary to demonstrate that guidelines are based on scientific evidence, all national guidelines are, by necessity, very lengthy documents. Although these national documents are intended to help primary care physicians in the everyday management of patients with CAP, in reality these very extensive documents are unlikely to be read by the audience they are intended for. It is also important to recognize that several aspects of care recommended in national guidelines as ideal care are based not on scientific evidence but on expert opinion. Then, a particular aspect of patient management suggested in a national guideline may not represent the recommended care proposed by the pneumonia team at the local hospital level.

In an attempt to correct some of the weaknesses of the national guidelines, the first task of the hospital multidisciplinary pneumonia team is to write a document for local recommended care that is concise and takes into account local factors. Some of the recommendations from national guidelines can be adapted to the local reality. This process will increase the local acceptability of the guideline.

The local hospital document needs to address only areas of practice that have a considerable impact on outcome and can be potentially improved by modification of local care. Antimicrobial therapy is one example of an area of practice that will have a significant impact on outcome and that can be potentially improved at the local hospital.

National guidelines usually have sections dedicated to the epidemiology of pneumonia or sections dedicated to delineating the clinical characteristics of patients infected with specific pathogens. These types of sections in the national guidelines are of almost no relevance to the day-to-day management of hospitalized patients with CAP and should not be addressed in the local hospital document.

Areas of Practice with High Impact on Outcome

The primary goal of implementing a local CAP guideline is to improve outcomes. The local care given to the hospitalized patient with CAP will have an impact over the patient's clinical outcome (e.g., clinical cure), patient-focused outcome (e.g., satisfaction with care), and economic outcome (e.g., resource utilization). Although a good outcome depends on all aspects of care, certain areas of patient management have a more direct effect on outcomes. The most common areas in the management of patients with CAP that will have a significant effect on patient outcomes, patient-focused outcomes, or economic outcomes are depicted in Figure 1.

Because these areas can be improved locally, there is the potential for local improvement of outcomes by modification of local practice of care. Not all areas of management need to be addressed in a local guideline document. The local team may want to develop a document with only a selected group of management areas in which changes in practice are likely to have a greater effect on outcomes. All local guidelines address the area of empiric antimicrobial therapy because the selection of appropriate antibiotics will have a significant impact on patients' clinical outcomes. Another commonly selected area of management is switch therapy, because an early switch from intravenous to oral antibiotic therapy will have a significant effect on economic outcome by decreasing the length of the patient's hospital stay.

Local Recommended Care

Once a series of practice areas has been selected, the local pneumonia team needs to clearly define for each selected area of management what will be the recommended local practice. This local recommended care should be translated into a clear statement that should be written so that it can have only one interpretation. It is important that every health care worker receive the same clear message after reading the statement of local recommended care. For example, a pneumonia guideline may have the following recommendation as the ideal time to switch patients to oral therapy: "Patients should be switched from intravenous to oral antibiotics when they are clinically stable." This type of statement for recommended care is likely to be interpreted differently by different physicians. Because when to consider a patient as be-

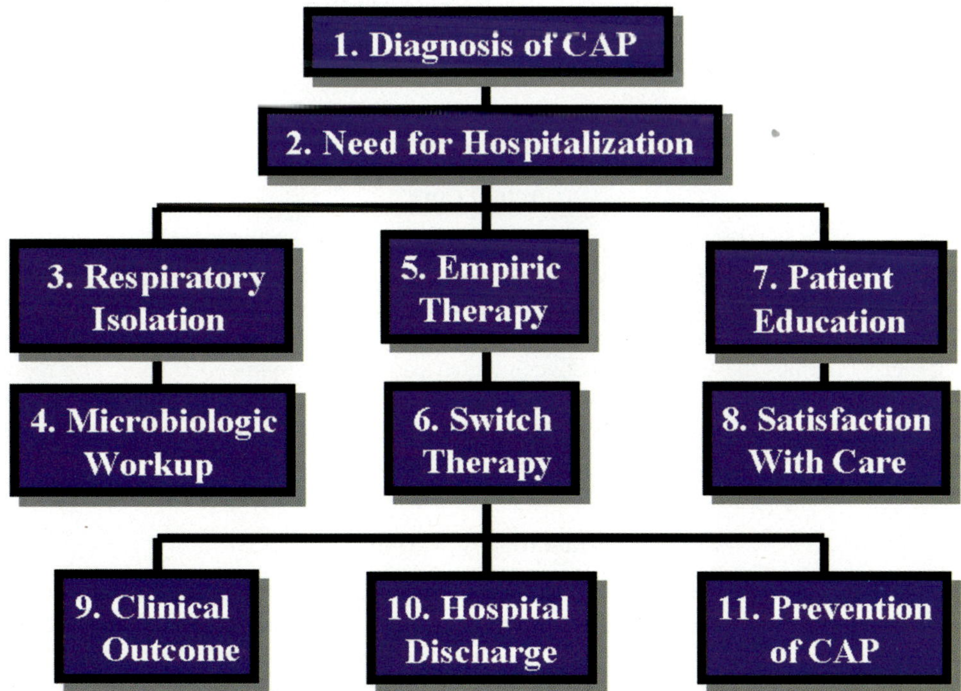

FIG. 1. Areas of patient management with high impact on outcomes. CAP, community-acquired pneumonia.

ing clinically stable is subject to personal interpretation, this type of local recommendation is likely to be associated with a significant variability among practitioners in the time to switch patients to oral therapy. It will be best for the local guideline to define clear and simple criteria of when a patient should be considered a candidate for switch therapy. The necessary background information to develop clear recommendations for local practice for each area of patient management is presented in subsequent chapters.

Quality Indicators

After defining the recommended care for a particular area of patient management, the team needs to evaluate what is the actual care in that particular area. To evaluate actual practice against recommended practice, the team should develop a list of quality indicators. A quality indicator is calculated as a percentage of the instances when recommended care was actually achieved divided by the instances in which recommended care was applicable. For example, a local hospital guideline recommends that hospitalized patients with CAP who present with risk factors for tuberculosis (TB), as described in the guideline document, should be admitted to an isolation room. A quality indicator regarding isolation of patients at risk for TB will be calculated as the percentage of patients placed in respiratory isolation divided by the total number of hospitalized patients with risk factors for TB.

Quality indicators to evaluate the management of hospitalized patients with CAP has been suggested by several national organizations such as the IDSA,[2] the Joint Commission on Accreditation of Healthcare Organizations (JCAHO),[6] the Center for Medicare and Medicaid Services (CMS),[7] and the American College of Physicians project for Assessing Care of Vulnerable Elders (ACOVE).[8] The selection of appropriate quality indicators of practice with clear numerators and denominators is an important step during the implementation of a practice guideline. In subsequent chapters, for each area of patient management, a list of suggested quality indicators is discussed.

STEP 2: COLLECTION AND EVALUATION OF DATA ON QUALITY INDICATORS

Actual Care

The data from the different quality indicators reflect the "actual care" delivered to a patient with CAP. It is important that the person responsible for data collection has a sufficient degree of expertise in the area to secure quality of the data. This step is facilitated with a clear and simple data collection form. The data collected should be used to generate reports in a format that clearly defines the difference between actual care and recommended care. The reports should also allow the comparison of actual care with recommended care over time. A computer database can greatly facilitate the generation of reports to evaluate quality of care over time. These reports can be used as a summary of clinical performance.

Evaluation of Variance

Variance can be defined as the difference or discrepancy between the recommended or planned care and what actually happened or actual care. Once data are collected and reports are generated, the team should have a clear view of the variance of actual care from recommended care. It should be emphasized that variance from recommended care does not necessarily imply poor clinical practice. It is important, after variance has been identified, to evaluate whether the variance should be considered clinically justified or unjustified.

Because a certain percentage of variance from recommended care will be expected for almost all quality indicators, the team may select a reasonable predetermined threshold of accepted variance. If this predetermined threshold is exceeded, evaluation of the data is performed to decide whether the variance was justified or unjustified. Evaluation of variance can be simplified by analyzing variance as related to (a) the health care worker, (b) the system, and (c) the patient.

Health Care Worker Variance

Health care worker variance occurs when a caregiver is unable to provide the care that is recommended in the guideline. Examples include a physician who prescribes an antibiotic that is not recommended in the local guideline or a nurse who failed to perform patient education on pneumonia.

System Variance

System variance occurs owing to a problem in the institution or health care system. Examples include the lack of availability of an isolation bed at the time that a patient with CAP and risk factors for tuberculosis is admitted to the hospital or a patient who was already switched to oral antibiotics and is ready for hospital discharge but needs to remain in the hospital owing to a delay in a diagnostic procedure (e.g., computed tomography [CT] scan, Holter).

Patient Variance

Patient variance occurs as a direct result of something the patient did or did not do. Examples include the need for hospitalization of a patient owing not to severity of pulmonary infection but to noncompliance with oral outpatient therapy.

STEP 3: INTERVENTIONS FOR IMPROVEMENT

Unjustified Variance

The pneumonia team should perform an intense analysis of all areas identified with unjustified variance because areas with unjustified variance are likely to be associated with poor outcomes. Once the root of unjustified variance is identified, the team will need to develop actions with the goal to decrease variance.

When poor quality of care is related to a system failure, it will be necessary to create the appropriate structural and organizational conditions to improve care. When poor quality of care is related to poor practice, it will be necessary to change local health care practices. It is recognized that from all health care workers, the most reluctant to change an established practice is the physician. Because several aspects of the management of the patient with CAP will depend on physicians' practices, the local pneumonia team will need to be aware of the possible interactions available to change local practice.

Changing Health Care Practice

In an attempt to change local health care practice, the pneumonia team will need to use a combination of interventions classified as follows:

Interventions before the Patient Is Hospitalized

Interventions before hospitalization include traditional education techniques such as lectures and courses given by local experts or national leaders in the field or the use of innovative educational tools such as computer programs with interactive learning.

Interventions during Patient Hospitalization

Types of interventions may occur while the patient is hospitalized: reminders of ideal practice and face-to-face interactions. Reminders of ideal practice can be placed by one of the members of the CAP team in the patient's medical record as a note attached to the record, without being an official part of the record, or a note on the daily progress note of the medical record. A face-to-face interaction of a member of the CAP team with the physician provides the opportunity to discuss the local recommended management. Interventions during hospitalization are considered very effective in changing practice. The problem is that this type of intervention requires that at least one member of the pneumonia team be able to provide a daily follow-up of all hospitalized patients with CAP. During this daily follow-up, the team member will have the opportunity to undergo a prospective evaluation of actual care and to identify variance in real time. With this type of intervention, a variance from recommended care can be recognized in a timely manner and acted on while the patient is still in the hospital.

Interventions after Hospitalization

After patients are discharged from the hospital, health care workers can receive feedback on their performance using the data from the local quality indicators. The feedback can be performed by reporting collective hospital data for all hospitalized patients with CAP. Another possibility is to report physician-specific data. If the pneumonia quality indicators are going to be used to generate physician-specific reports, it is important that evaluation of justified versus unjustified variance from recommended care is performed by a peer review committee.

STEP 4: RECOLLECTION AND EVALUATION OF DATA ON QUALITY INDICATORS

The last step in the process is the recollection of quality indicator data to evaluate whether variance was minimized or eliminated. A decrease in variance proves that practice has changed in the way desired. This on-going data collection is necessary to permit documentation of local improvement in the management of patients with CAP.

SUMMARY

The necessary steps for development and implementation of a national guideline at the hospital level are summarized in Figure 2. After the local multidisciplinary team suggests a recommended care, data are collected on actual care to define whether variance is present. If unjustified variance is identified, the team develops an intervention with the goal to move actual practice closer to the recommended practice. Data are collected and evaluated again to define whether variance was decreased. Documentation of decreased variance is necessary to prove that the local guideline is being successfully implemented.

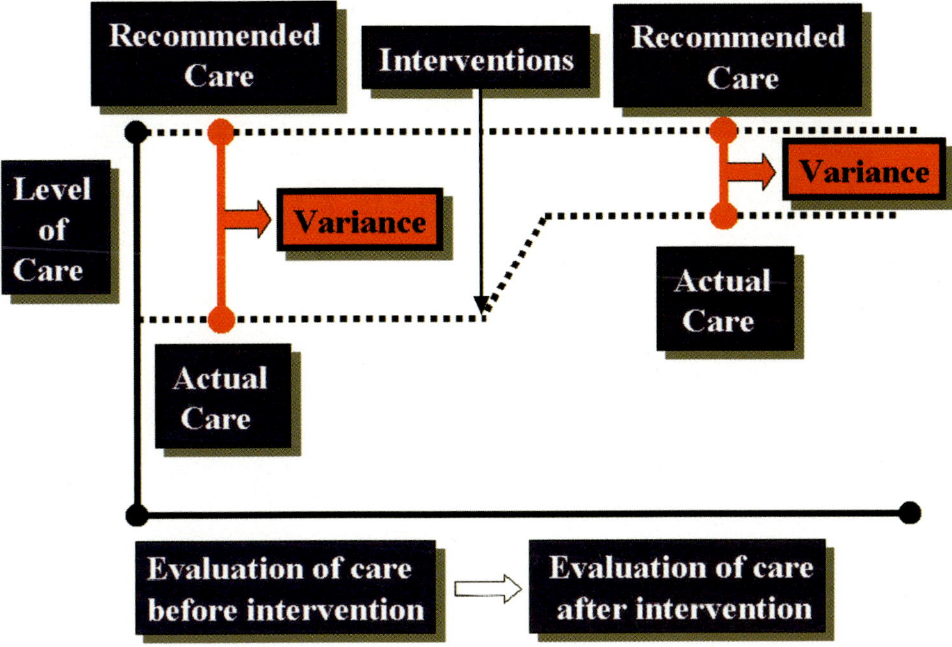

FIG. 2. Steps during local implementation of guidelines for treating community-acquired pneumonia.

REFERENCES

1. Niederman MS, Bass JB, Campbell GD, et al: Guidelines for the initial management of adults with community-acquired pneumonia: Diagnosis, assessment of severity, and initial antimicrobial therapy. *Am Rev Respir Dis* 1993;148:1418–1426.
2. Bartlett JG, Dowell SF, Mandell LA, et al: Practice guidelines for the management of community-acquired pneumonia in adults. Guidelines from the Infectious Diseases Society of America. *Clin Infect Dis* 2000;31: 347–382.
3. Heffelfinger JD, Dowell SF, Jorgensen JH, et al: Management of community-acquired pneumonia in the era of pneumococcal resistance: a report from the Drug-Resistant *Streptococcus pneumoniae* Therapeutic Working Group. *Arch Intern Med* 2000;160:1399–1408.
4. American College of Emergency Physicians. Clinical policy for the management and risk stratification of community-acquired pneumonia in adults in the emergency department. *Ann Emerg Med* 2001;38:107–113.
5. Niederman MS, Mandell LA, Anzueto A, et al;. Guidelines for the management of adults with community-acquired pneumonia. American Thoracic Society. *Am J Respir Crit Care Med* 2001;163:1730–1754.
6. Plan for Introducing Joint Commission Hospital Core Measure Requirements. http://www.jcaho.org/perfmeas/coremeas/core_manual.htm
7. Department of Health and Human Services Health Care Financing Administration: Operational Policy Letter no. 116, OPL2000.116. http://www.hcfa.gov/medicare/opl116.htm
8. Rhew DC: Quality indicators for the management of pneumonia in vulnerable elders. *Ann Intern Med* 2001;135:736–743.

2

Clinical Diagnosis of Pneumonia

Pneumonia Pathogenesis
The Pneumonia Syndrome
Clinical Diagnosis
Evaluation of Local Practice
Quality Indicator
Proportion of Patients Who Met Diagnostic Criteria of Community-Acquired Pneumonia
Evaluation of Variance from Recommended Care
References

PNEUMONIA PATHOGENESIS

Pneumonia indicates an inflammatory process of the lung parenchyma that is caused by a microbial agent. The most common pathway for the microbial agent to reach the alveoli is by microaspiration of oropharyngeal secretions. Once microorganisms reach the alveolar space, they cause pneumonia by overcoming the last defense mechanism of the lung, the alveolar macrophage. Most of the time, the alveolar macrophage phagocytizes and kills the microorganisms that reach the alveolar space. This explains why even though the arrival of microorganisms into the alveolar space is a not-infrequent occurrence, the presence of clinical pneumonia is infrequent (Fig. 1).

If the alveolar macrophage is unable to control the growth of the microorganisms, then, as a final protective defense mechanism, the lungs develop a local inflammatory response. This local inflammatory response is characterized by movement of white blood cells, lymphocytes, and monocytes from the capillaries into the alveolar space (Fig. 2).

The recruitment of phagocytic cells to the alveolar space is primarily mediated by tumor necrosis factor (TNF) and interleukin-1 (IL-1) produced by the alveolar macrophages. In addition to TNF and IL-1, other important locally produced cytokines include IL-6, IL-10, IL-12, monocyte chemotaxin protein–1, and granulocyte colony–stimulating factor.[1] Once these cytokines reach the systemic circulation, they also produce a systemic inflammatory response. The local and systemic inflammatory response is responsible for the majority of the signs, symptoms, and laboratory abnormalities that characterize the community-acquired pneumonia (CAP) syndrome.

THE PNEUMONIA SYNDROME

The patient with pneumonia syndrome will present with cough, sputum production, shortness of breath, pleuritic chest pain, fever, chills, tachycardia, tachypnea, rales, and signs of consolidation on physical examination, leukocytosis, left shift, and a new pulmonary infiltrate on chest x-ray. Several of these abnormalities are due to the local inflammatory response pro-

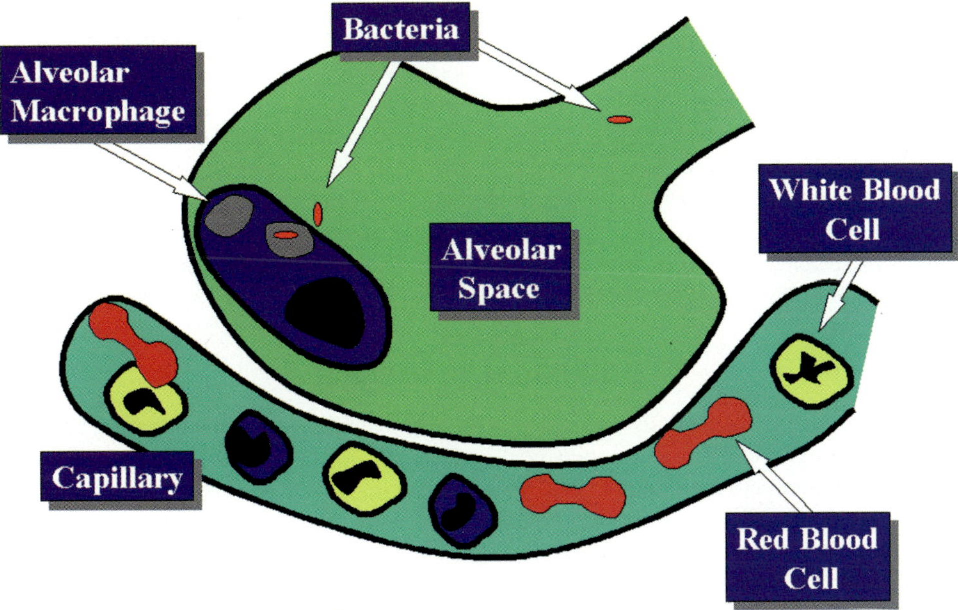

FIG. 1. The alveolar macrophage acting as a last-defense mechanism against bacteria that reach the alveolar space.

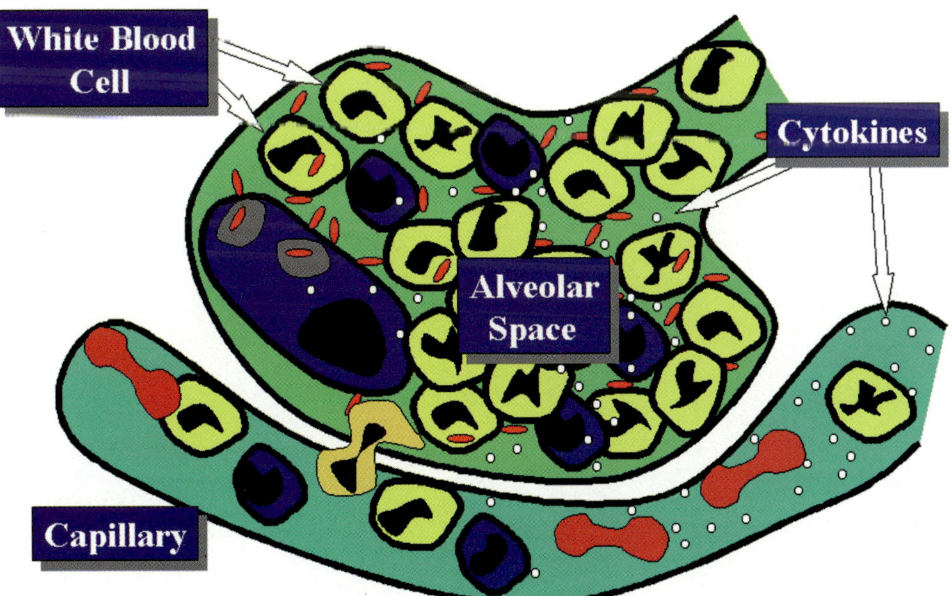

FIG. 2. Recruitment of phagocytic cells to the alveolar space mediated by the local production of cytokines.

duced by the arrival of white blood cells into the alveolar space. The development of cough and sputum production are due to the excess of white blood cells in the alveoli. The shortness of breath and hypoxemia are secondary to the accumulation of cells in the alveolar space, producing a ventilation-perfusion mismatching. The presence of a new pulmonary infiltrate at chest x-ray is predominantly due to the buildup of inflammatory cells in the alveoli (Fig. 3).

Other manifestations of the pneumonia syndrome are due to the systemic inflammatory response. The presence of fever is primarily mediated by the action of IL-1 and other mediators that act on the thermoregulatory center at the level of the hypothalamus. The presence of leukocytosis and left shift is primarily mediated by the action of granulocyte colony–stimulating factor on the bone marrow (Fig. 3).

CLINICAL DIAGNOSIS

Owing to the low sensitivity and specificity, history and physical examination are considered suboptimal to confirm or exclude the diagnosis of CAP.[2] National guidelines recommend that a new pulmonary infiltrate at chest x-ray should be present to classify a hospitalized patient as having the diagnosis of CAP.[3,4] The clinical diagnosis requires evidence of a new pulmonary infiltrate compatible with pneumonia associated with other signs and symptoms characteristic of the pneumonia syndrome. Because the clinical diagnosis of CAP is based on a clinical syndrome, it is expected that in some hospitalized patients with a clinical diagnosis of CAP, an alternative diagnosis will explain the signs and symptoms of the patient. Although the patient may have cough, sputum production, and fever, sometimes the infection represents not pneumonia but an acute exacerbation of chronic bronchitis or acute bronchitis. In this type of patient, there will be no evidence of a new pulmonary infiltrate. In patients with a pulmonary infiltrate at admission to the hospital, the infiltrate may be not a new infiltrate but a chronic one representing old pulmonary changes. In some patients with a new pulmonary infiltrate, it may be due to an alternative diagnosis such as pulmonary embolism. In a study performed in our institution, we found that the most common clinical scenario associated with a

Local Inflammatory Response
+ Cough
+ Sputum
+ Chest pain
+ Tachypnea
+ Dyspnea
+ Rales
+ Pulmonary infiltrate
Systemic Inflammatory Response
+ Fever
+ Tachycardia
+ Malaise
+ Anorexia
+ Leukocytosis
+ Left shift
+ Hypothermia
+ Neutropenia

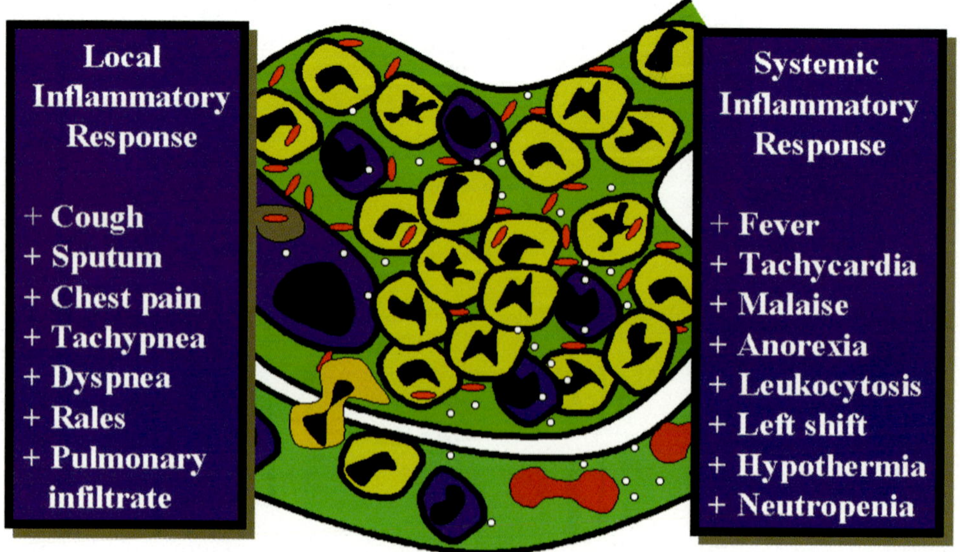

FIG. 3. The clinical and laboratory manifestations of the pneumonia syndrome according to the local or the systemic inflammatory response.

misdiagnosis of CAP is the patient admitted to hospital with cough and a new pulmonary infiltrate due to an exacerbation of congestive heart failure.[5]

EVALUATION OF LOCAL PRACTICE

The diagnosis of CAP can be selected as an area for evaluation of local practice. In our institution, patients meet guideline criteria for CAP when they present with a new pulmonary infiltrate at hospital admission, associated with at least one of the following: (a) new or increased cough, (b) fever or hypothermia, and (c) leukocytosis, left shift, or neutropenia. A sample form to collect data on quality indicators for the evaluation of this area of practice can be found in the Appendix. A current update of the literature in this area of practice can be found at www.caposite.com.

QUALITY INDICATOR

Proportion of Patients Who Met Diagnostic Criteria of Community-Acquired Pneumonia

The proportion of patients who met diagnostic criteria for CAP according to local guidelines can be used as a quality indicator. For this indicator the numerator will be the total number of patients that met diagnostic criteria of CAP, and the denominator, the total number of patients hospitalized with diagnosis of CAP according to primary physician. The goal is to improve quality by preventing errors in the diagnosis of CAP, since patients with an alternative diagnosis will not benefit from the management suggested for patients with CAP.

EVALAUTION OF VARIANCE FROM RECOMMENDED CARE

A patient with diagnosis of CAP without a new pulmonary infiltrate is considered to have a justified variance from recommended care if the patient has severe neutropenia, acquired immunodeficiency syndrome (AIDS), or dehydration. Any of these conditions may produce a clinical picture of CAP with a pulmonary infiltrate that may not be evident during the initial chest radiograph. In the immunocompromised host with CAP, a pulmonary infiltrate that is not detected by a chest x-ray can be seen using computed tomography of the chest.[6] Patients with a diagnosis of CAP without a new pulmonary infiltrate and without any of the conditions described previously is considered to have an unjustified variance from recommended care. Another reason for unjustified variance is the presence of an infiltrate that is not acute but chronic.

It is important to differentiate patients with CAP from those with hospital-acquired pneumonia because the likely organisms and appropriate empiric therapy are different. Patients hospitalized with a diagnosis of CAP that, according to our local guidelines, met the diagnosis of nosocomial pneumonia, are considered to have an incorrect diagnosis of CAP with unjustified variance. In our guidelines, pneumonia is considered nosocomial instead of community-acquired in patients who develop pneumonia after 72 hours of hospitalization. In patients who were recently hospitalized and developed pneumonia at home, controversy exists regarding the number of days that the patient needs to be at home before the pneumonia is characterized as community-acquired. Our guidelines define pneumonia as community-acquired if it develops after the patient has been at home for 14 days. Prior to 14 days, the pneumonia is classified as nosocomial. A caveat of this definition is that the patient must be in the hospital for more than 3 days to meet the definition of prior hospitalization. Any hospitalization of 3 days or less is not considered a risk factor for the acquisition of nosocomial pathogens.

REFERENCES

1. Nelson S, Mason CM, Kolls J, Summer WR: Pathophysiology of pneumonia. *Clin Chest Med* 1995;16:1–123.
2. Wipf JE, Lipsky BA, Hirschmann JV, et al: Diagnosing pneumonia by physical examination: relevant or relic? *Arch Intern Med* 1999;159:1082–1087.
3. Niederman MS, Mandell LA, Anzueto A, et al: Guidelines for the management of adults with community-acquired pneumonia. American Thoracic Society. *Am J Respir Crit Care Med* 2001;163: 1730–1754.
4. Bartlett JG, Dowell SF, Mandell LA, et al: Practice guidelines for the management of community-acquired pneumonia in adults. Guidelines from the Infectious Diseases Society of America. *Clin Infect Dis* 2000;31:347–382.
5. Ahkee S, Barzallo M, Ramirez J: Empiric antibiotic therapy in patients without documented infections. *Infect Med* 1996;13:800–802, 823.
6. Wheeler JH, Fishman EK: Computed tomography in the management of chest infections: current status. *Clin Infect Dis* 1996;23:232–240.

3

Need for Hospitalization

Site of Care
Hospitalization Based on Patient's Risk for Complicated Course
Hospitalization Based on Patient's Risk for Mortality
Hospital Admission Decision
Evaluation of Local Practice
Quality Indicators
Proportion of Patients Hospitalized with Risk Classes III to V • Proportion of Patients Hospitalized with More than 1 Criteria for Complicated Course
Evaluation of Variance from Recommended Care
References

SITE OF CARE

During the initial evaluation of the patient with community-acquired pneumonia (CAP), the physician needs to define the patient's severity of disease and the intensity of care that will be necessary for the patient to achieve an optimal outcome. If the level of care the patient can receive at home is not sufficient, the patient will require hospitalization.

Hospitalization will permit the use of intravenous antibiotics, intravenous fluids, hemodynamic support, supplemental oxygen, mechanical ventilation, and aggressive therapy of comorbidity and will facilitate several clinical evaluations performed by nurses and physicians during the day.

HOSPITALIZATION BASED ON PATIENT'S RISK FOR COMPLICATED COURSE

In an attempt to help physicians in the evaluation of patient's severity of disease and risk for mortality, the American Thoracic Society published a list of criteria associated with poor outcome in patients with CAP (Table 1).[1]

The document indicates that hospitalization can be based on the number of criteria for complicated course identified in a patient. It is suggested that a patient with more than one criteria for complicated course will benefit from hospitalization.

HOSPITALIZATION BASED ON PATIENT'S RISK FOR MORTALITY

A prediction rule to identify low-risk patients with CAP was derived using data from 14,199 adults with CAP.[2] To parallel physician decision-making processes, the prediction rule was developed in two steps.

TABLE 1. *Risk factors associated with a complicated course of community-acquired pneumonia*

Demographic	Comorbid illness	Signs and symptoms	Laboratory findings	Chest x-ray findings
Age > 65 yr Nursing home resident	COPD, CHF, diabetes, neoplasia, ETOH, chronic renal failure, liver disease, aspiration, neurologic disease, post splenectomy, immunosuppression, prior admission for CAP within 1 yr	RR > 30, HR > 125, T < 95 or > 104 Diastolic BP < 60 mm/Hg Systolic BP < 90 mm/Hg Abnormal mental status Extrapulmonary site of infection	WBC < 4K, or > 20K, or ANC < 1K BUN > 30, Creatinine > 1.2 mg Hct < 30%, Hg < 9 mg/dl Albumin < 2.6 g/L Na < 130 mEq/L Platelet < 100 K Glucose > 250 mg/dl Po_2 < 60, or Pao_2/Fio_2 < 300, or O_2 Sat < 90% Pco_2 > 50 pH < 7.35 Need for mechanical ventilation Bacteremia	Multiple lobe involvement Presence of a cavity Pleural effusion

ANC, absolute neutrophil count; BP, blood pressure; BUN, Blood urea nitrogen; CAP, community-acquired pneumonia; CHF, congestive heart failure; COPD, chronic obstructive pulmonary disease; ETOH, alcohol abuse; Fio_2, fraction of inspired oxygen; Hct, hematocrit; Hg, hemoglobin; HR, heart rate; O_2 Sat, oxygen saturation; Pao_2, partial pressure of oxygen, arterial; Pco_2, partial pressure of carbon dioxide; Po_2, partial pressure of oxygen; RR, respiratory rate; WBC, white blood count.

From Niederman MS, Mandell LA, Anzueto A, et al: Guidelines for the management of adults with community-acquired pneumonia. American Thoracic Society. Am J Respir Crit Care Med 2001;163: 1730–1754, with permission.

Step 1. This step identified a subgroup of patients at low risk of death solely on the basis of their history and physical examination findings. These patients are classified as class I (Table 2).

Step 2. The risk of death was quantified in the remaining patients with the same 11 findings used in step 1 plus 2 demographic factors and 7 laboratory or radiographic findings. A scoring system was used to measure the magnitude of association of these factors with mortality and to assign patients a total number of points (Table 3).

Based on the total points assigned, patients are classified in risk class II (≤70 points), risk class III (71–90 points), risk class IV (91–130 points), or risk class V (>130 points). Among the different classes, the mortality rate is 0.1 percent for class I patients, 0.6 percent for class II patients, 2.8 percent for class III patients, 8.2 percent for class IV patients, and 29.2 percent for class V patients.

Patients 50 years of age or younger who have none of the coexisting illnesses or physical findings identified as class I are considered candidates for outpatient treatment. Importantly, physicians can make this determination on the basis of information obtained from the initial history and physical examination without having to order laboratory tests, which may be costly and time-consuming. Patients assigned to risk class II are considered candidates for outpatient therapy. Patients assigned to risk class III, IV, or V are considered candidates for hospitalization. The national guidelines of the Infectious Diseases Society of America (IDSA) support the use of this prediction rule to assist with the decision of hospitalization.[3]

TABLE 2. *Step one of the pneumonia severity index*

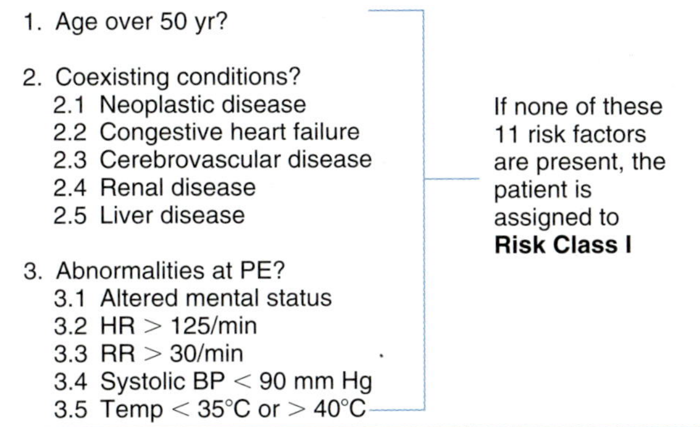

1. Age over 50 yr?
2. Coexisting conditions?
   - 2.1 Neoplastic disease
   - 2.2 Congestive heart failure
   - 2.3 Cerebrovascular disease
   - 2.4 Renal disease
   - 2.5 Liver disease
3. Abnormalities at PE?
   - 3.1 Altered mental status
   - 3.2 HR > 125/min
   - 3.3 RR > 30/min
   - 3.4 Systolic BP < 90 mm Hg
   - 3.5 Temp < 35°C or > 40°C

If none of these 11 risk factors are present, the patient is assigned to **Risk Class I**

BP, blood pressure; HR, heart rate; PE, physical examination; RR, respiratory rate.

From Fine MJ, Auble TE, Yealy DM, et al: A prediction rule to identify low-risk patients with community-acquired pneumonia. N Engl J Med 1997;336:243–250, with permission.

HOSPITAL ADMISSION DECISION

Even with the availability of risk stratification data, the admission decision is ultimately an art-of-medicine decision, which should be carefully individualized. Nonclinical factors, such as patient preference, and social considerations, including insurance and reimbursement issues, may also influence the site-of-care decision.

It is important to keep in mind that the decision to hospitalize is not necessarily a commitment to long-term inpatient care. Rather, it is a decision that certain patients should be observed closely until it is evident that their infection is responding to therapy.

EVALUATION OF LOCAL PRACTICE

The need for hospitalization can be selected as an area for evaluation of local practice. In our institution, patients meet guideline criteria for appropriate hospitalization if (a) they were

TABLE 3. *Point score according to patient's characteristics*

1. Demographic factor age		4. Physical examination findings	
Men	Age (yr)	Altered mental status	+20
Women	Age (yr) − 10	Respiratory rate > 30	+20
		Systolic BP < 90	+20
2. Nursing home resident		Temperature < 35° or > 40°C	+15
	+ 10	Pulse > 125	+10
3. Coexisting conditions		5. Laboratory and x-ray findings	
Neoplastic disease	+30	Arterial pH < 7.35	+30
Liver disease	+20	BUN > 30 mg/dl	+20
Congestive heart failure	+10	Sodium < 130 mmol/L	+20
Cerebrovascular disease	+10	Glucose > 250 mg/dl	+10
Renal disease	+10	Hematocrit < 30%	+10
		Pao_2 < 60 mmHg	+10
		Pleural effusion	+10

BP, blood pressure; BUN, blood urea nitrogen; Pao_2, partial pressure of oxygen, arterial.

stratified to a risk class III, IV, or V, or (b) they had more than one risk factor for complicated course. A sample form to collect data on quality indicators for the evaluation of this area of practice can be found in the Appendix. A current update of the literature in this area of practice can be found at www.caposite.com.

QUALITY INDICATORS

Proportion of Patients Hospitalized with Risk Classes III to V

The proportion of patients with appropriate hospitalization according to risk class can be used as a quality indicator. For this indicator, the numerator is the total number of patients hospitalized with risk class III, IV, or V, and the denominator is the total number of hospitalized patients who met diagnostic criteria for CAP. The goal is to improve quality by preventing unnecessary hospitalization.

Proportion of Patients Hospitalized with More than 1 Criteria for Complicated Course

The proportion of patients with appropriate hospitalization according to number of risk factors for complicated course can be used as a quality indicator. For this indicator, the numerator is the total number of patients hospitalized with more than 1 criteria for complicated course, and the denominator is the total number of hospitalized patients who met diagnostic criteria for CAP. The goal is to improve quality by preventing unnecessary hospitalization.

EVALUATION OF VARIANCE FROM RECOMMENDED CARE

Patients who do not fulfill criteria for hospitalization because they are classified as risk class I or II, or who have no criteria for complicated course, may still have a reason for justified hospitalization. Admission may be justified in patients who (a) are unable to take oral antibiotics owing to nausea or vomiting, (b) failed outpatient therapy, (c) have social needs, (d) have suspected sepsis, or (e) do not have severe CAP but require admission owing to deterioration of comorbidity.

REFERENCES

1. Niederman MS, Mandell LA, Anzueto A, et al: Guidelines for the management of adults with community-acquired pneumonia. American Thoracic Society. *Am J Respir Crit Care Med* 2001;163: 1730–1754.
2. Fine MJ, Auble TE, Yealy DM, et al: A prediction rule to identify low-risk patients with community-acquired pneumonia. *N Engl J Med* 1997;336:243–250.
3. Bartlett JG, Dowell SF, Mandell LA, et al: Practice guidelines for the management of community-acquired pneumonia in adults. Guidelines from the Infectious Diseases Society of America. *Clin Infect Dis* 2000;31:347–382.

4
Respiratory Isolation

Tuberculosis Presenting as Community-Acquired Pneumonia
Tuberculosis Presenting as Chronic Community-Acquired Pneumonia • Tuberculosis Presenting as Acute Community-Acquired Pneumonia
Respiratory Isolation
Evaluation of Local Practice
Quality Indicators
Proportion of Patients Placed in Respiratory Isolation • Proportion of Patients with Acid-fast Bacilli Smears and Culture Obtained on Day 1 • Proportion of Patients with Isolation Discontinued after Only Two Negative Acid-fast Bacilli Smears
Evaluation of Variance from Recommended Care
References

TUBERCULOSIS PRESENTING AS COMMUNITY-ACQUIRED PNEUMONIA

Pneumonia can be classified according to the duration of signs and symptoms as acute or chronic. A patient with a pulmonary infiltrate and duration of pulmonary symptoms for weeks, rather than days, is considered to have chronic pneumonia.[1] In our institution, patients who present with less than 14 days of pulmonary signs and symptoms are considered to have acute community-acquired pneumonia (CAP). Patients who present with more than 2 weeks of signs and symptoms are considered to have chronic CAP. A patient with pulmonary tuberculosis (TB) may present with a clinical syndrome of acute or chronic CAP.

Tuberculosis Presenting as Chronic Community-Acquired Pneumonia

Pulmonary TB is classically suspected in patients that present with several weeks of cough, sputum production with hemoptysis, fever, night sweats, loss of weight, and a pulmonary infiltrate involving the upper lobes of the lung. This presentation of chronic pneumonia is the most common clinical presentation for patients with pulmonary TB. This form of pulmonary TB is usually due to the reactivation of an old tuberculous granuloma of the lung that developed several years earlier, during the patientís primary TB infection.

Tuberculosis Presenting as Acute Community-Acquired Pneumonia

When TB pneumonia develops during primary TB infection, the patient may present with a syndrome of acute CAP.[2] The patient has less than 14 days of signs and symptoms with fever, cough, and a new pulmonary infiltrate. Because primary TB infection usually develops in the lower lobes, the patient presents with a clinical picture of acute pneumonia with a lobar lower lobe pulmonary infiltrate. The clinical presentation of a patient with acute pulmonary TB can be indistinguishable from the clinical presentation of a patient with a common bacterial pneumonia such as pneumococcal pneumonia.

RESPIRATORY ISOLATION

Because TB can present with a clinical picture of acute or chronic pneumonia, a high index of suspicion for TB should be maintained in all hospitalized patients with a clinical diagnosis of CAP. All patients admitted for CAP should be screened to define whether the patient has risk factors for pulmonary TB. Risk factors for pulmonary TB according to the Centers for Disease Control and Prevention are presented in Table 1.[3] Some of the risk factors described in Table 1 are associated with an increased risk for acquisition of the disease (e.g., recent exposure to a patient with active TB); others are associated with an increased risk of developing active disease in patients who were previously exposed and have latent disease or who are otherwise immunocompromised (e.g., receiving long-term cortisone therapy). Patients admitted to hospital with CAP and one or more risk factors for TB should be considered to have active pulmonary TB until proved otherwise. Patients with CAP who have risk factors for TB should be admitted to the hospital and placed in respiratory isolation until TB has been ruled out. These patients should be admitted to an isolation room to protect other patients as well as health care personnel.

Sputum for acid-fast bacilli (AFB) smears and culture should be obtained without delay in patients with suspicion of TB. A rapid confirmation of the diagnosis benefits the patient by allowing rapid initiation of treatment. A rapid exclusion of the diagnosis allows rapid discontinuation of isolation. If clinically indicated, a purified protein derivative (PPD) skin test with control should be obtained on the day of admission to the hospital.

Based on national recommendations, most hospitals isolate patients in whom tuberculosis is suspected until three smear results are negative. But considering our experience and recent

TABLE 1. *Risk factors associated with tuberculosis*

Signs and symptoms	Member of high risk group	History of chronic illness
Night sweats	HIV-positive	End-stage renal disease
Hemoptysis	History of positive PPD	Cancer of the mouth or GI tract
Weight loss	Homeless	Diabetes
Hoarseness	Age > 65 yr	Hematologic disease
	Alcohol or drug abuse	Gastrectomy
	Health care worker	Chronic malabsorption syndrome
	History of TB	Intestinal bypass
	Recent exposure to active TB	Silicosis
	Community living (prison, nursing home, shelter)	Less than 10% of ideal body weight
	Immigrant (Asia, Africa, or South America)	Long-term cortisone therapy
		Other immunosuppressive state

GI, gastrointestinal; HIV, human immunodeficiency virus; PPD, purified protein derivative; TB, tuberculosis.

Core Curriculum on Tuberculosis. What the Clinician Should Know, 4th ed. Atlanta, US Department of Health and Human Services, Centers for Disease Control and Prevention, National Center for HIV, STD, and TB prevention, Division of Tuberculosis Elimination, 2000, with permission.

reports in the literature, the need for the third negative smear is questionable. In patients suspected of having TB with the first two smears negative, the third smear will be also negative.[4,5]

EVALUATION OF LOCAL PRACTICE

The management of patients at risk for TB can be selected as an area for evaluation of local practice. In our institution, patients with CAP and at least one risk factor for TB are considered to have appropriate management when (a) the patient was admitted to respiratory isolation, (b) AFB smears and culture were obtained on day 1, and (c) the patient was removed from isolation when at least two negative AFB smears were documented. A sample form to collect data on quality indicators for the evaluation of this area of practice can be found in the Appendix. A current update of the literature in this area of practice can be found at www.caposite.com.

QUALITY INDICATORS

Proportion of Patients Placed in Respiratory Isolation

The proportion of patients placed in respiratory isolation can be used as a quality indicator. For this indicator, the numerator is the total number of patients placed on isolation, and the denominator is the total number of patients at risk for pulmonary TB. The goal is to improve quality by preventing nosocomial transmission of TB.

Proportion of Patients with Acid-fast Bacilli Smears and Culture Obtained on Day 1

The proportion of patients with AFB smears and culture obtained on day 1 can be used as a quality indicator. For this indicator, the numerator is the total number of patients with AFB smears and culture obtained on day 1, and the denominator is the total number of patients placed on respiratory isolation. The goal is to improve quality by achieving early diagnosis and therapy of patients with TB.

Proportion of Patients with Isolation Discontinued after Only Two Negative Acid-fast Bacilli Smears

The proportion of patients with isolation discontinued after only two negative AFB smears have been documented can be used as a quality indicator. For this indicator, the numerator is the total number of patients with respiratory isolation discontinued after documentation of only two negative AFB smears, and the denominator is the total number of patients placed on respiratory isolation. The goal is to improve quality by preventing early discontinuation of isolation in patients in whom TB has not been adequately ruled out.

EVALUATION OF VARIANCE FROM RECOMMENDED CARE

No reason can justify the lack of respiratory isolation in a hospitalized patient with CAP and risk factors for pulmonary TB. Once a patient is in isolation, the lack of a sample for AFB smear and culture on day 1 may have a justified reason in the patient who is not able to produce sputum.

Discontinuation of isolation even before the results of two negative AFB smears are known can be justified when an alternative etiology for CAP is identified before TB has been ruled out. The most common example is the patient admitted with CAP, placed on isolation because of the presence of risk factors for TB, with positive blood cultures for *Streptococcus pneumoniae* during the first day of hospitalization. In this patient, it is justified to discontinue isolation after documentation of a bacterial etiology for CAP even though two negative AFB smears have not been documented.

REFERENCES

1. Dismukes WE: Chronic pneumonia. In Mandell GL, Bennett JE, Dolin R (eds): *Mandell, Douglas, and Bennett's Principles and Practice of Infectious Diseases,* 5th ed. Philadelphia, WB Saunders, 2000; Chap. 60, pp. 755–767
2. Glassroth J: Tuberculosis. In Niederman MS, Sarosi GA, Glassroth J (eds): *Respiratory Infections,* 2nd ed. Philadelphia, Lippincott Williams & Wilkins, 2001; Chap. 37, pp. 475–486.
3. Core Curriculum on Tuberculosis. *What the Clinician Should Know*, 4th ed. Atlanta, US Department of Health and Human Services, Centers for Disease Control and Prevention, National Center for HIV, STD, and TB Prevention, Division of Tuberculosis Elimination, 2000.
4. Craft DW, Jones MC, Blanchet CN, Hopfer RL: Value of examining three acid-fast bacillus sputum smears for removal of patients suspected of having tuberculosis from the "airborne precautions" category. *J Clin Microbio.* 2000;38:4285–4287.
5. Siddiqui AH, Perl TM, Conlon M, et al: Preventing nosocomial transmission of pulmonary tuberculosis: when may isolation be discontinued for patients with suspected tuberculosis? *Infect Control Hosp Epidemiol* 2002;23:141–144.

5

Microbiologic Workup

Etiology of Community-Acquired Pneumonia
The Importance of Defining the Etiology of Community-Acquired Pneumonia
Laboratory Workup
Evaluation of Local Practice
Quality Indicators
Proportion of Patients with Sputum Gram Stain and Culture Available in Less than 72 Hours • Proportion of Patients with Blood Culture Result Available in Less than 72 Hours • Proportion of Patients with Blood Culture Obtained before Administration of Antibiotic
Evaluation of Variance from Recommended Care
References

ETIOLOGY OF COMMUNITY-ACQUIRED PNEUMONIA

In clinical studies designed to identify the etiology of CAP, using reference microbiology laboratories, a specific pathogen is not identified in approximately 50 percent of the patients.[1,2] In everyday practice, clinicians are expected to encounter pneumonia of unknown etiology in more than half of the hospitalized patients with community acquired pnuemonia (CAP). The etiology of CAP can be classified into four groups: (a) CAP caused by typical or conventional bacteria, (b) CAP caused by atypical bacteria, (c) CAP caused by other agents, and (d) CAP of unknown etiology. The incidence of the most common organisms causing CAP, according to a review of the international literature performed by the author, is presented in Table 1.

THE IMPORTANCE OF DEFINING THE ETIOLOGY OF COMMUNITY-ACQUIRED PNEUMONIA

Defining the etiology of pneumonia may have significant implications for patient management. In patients who are clinically improving after initiation of broad-spectrum empiric therapy, knowing the etiology may allow streamlining the regimen with therapy directed to the identified pathogen. Antibiotic streamlining may prevent selection of resistant bacteria and decrease cost of therapy. In the hospitalized patient with pneumonia who suffers clinical deterioration after initial empiric therapy, defining the etiology of pneumonia may explain the reason for the deterioration, help in the selection of alternative therapy, and improve clinical outcome. Other potential benefits of defining the etiology of CAP include the appropriate isolation of patients infected with pathogens that can be transmitted to other patients or health care personnel (e.g., *Mycobacterium tuberculosis*, influenza virus).

TABLE 1. *Incidence of the common etiologies of community-acquired pneumonia*

1. Typical pathogens	40%–60%
Streptococcus pneumoniae	15%–25%
Haemophilus influenzae	2%–10%
Moraxella catharralis	0%–5%
2. Atypical pathogens	10%–30%
Mycoplasma pneumoniae	1%–10%
Chlamydia pneumoniae	5%–15%
Legionella pneumophila	0%–15%
3. Other pathogens	5%–25%
Viral agents	2%–15%
Pneumocystis carinii	0%–10%
Mycobacterium tuberculosis	0%–10%
4. Unknown etiology	30%–60%

LABORATORY WORKUP

In an attempt to determine whether a typical pathogen is the etiology of pneumonia, it is recommended that all patients should have a sputum specimen for Gram stain and culture as well as two sets of blood cultures obtained before the institution of antimicrobial therapy.[1,2] The quality of sputum specimen should be determined by Gram stain results. Only sputum specimens that contain good numbers of leukocytes and minimal numbers of epithelial cells per low-power field should be accepted for bacterial culture. Most national guidelines consider that a sputum sample for Gram stain, culture and sensitivity, and blood cultures should be obtained in all hospitalized patients. The Infectious Diseases Society of America (IDSA) recommends the urinary antigen test for detection of *Legionella pneumophila* in patients with severe CAP who are hospitalized in the intensive care unit (ICU).[2]

EVALUATION OF LOCAL PRACTICE

The microbiologic workup to define etiology can be selected as an area for evaluation of local practice. In our institution, patients meet guideline criteria for basic microbiologic workup when (a) the result of sputum Gram stain and culture were available during the first 72 hours, (b) the result of two sets of blood cultures were available during the first 72 hours, and (c) the two sets of blood cultures were obtained before the first dose of antibiotic was administered. A sample form to collect data on quality indicators for the evaluation of this area of practice can be found in the Appendix. A current update of the literature in this area of practice can be found at www.caposite.com.

QUALITY INDICATORS

Proportion of Patients with Sputum Gram Stain and Culture Available in Less than 72 Hours

The proportion of patients with sputum Gram stain and culture available in less than 72 hours after hospitalization can be used as a quality indicator. For this indicator, the numerator is the total number of patients with sputum Gram stain and culture available in less than 72 hours after admission, and the denominator is the total number of patients who met diagnostic criteria for CAP. The goal is to improve quality by early determination of the etiology of CAP.

Proportion of Patients with Blood Culture Result Available in Less than 72 Hours

The proportion of patients with blood culture result available in less than 72 hours after hospitalization can be used as a quality indicator. For this indicator, the numerator is the total number of patients with blood culture available in less than 72 hours, and the denominator is the total number of patients who met diagnostic criteria for CAP. The goal is to improve quality by early determination of the etiology of CAP.

Proportion of Patients with Blood Culture Obtained before Administration of Antibiotic

The proportion of patients with blood culture obtained before administration of antibiotic therapy can be used as a quality indicator. For this indicator, the numerator is the total number of patients with blood culture obtained before administration of antibiotic, and the denominator is the total number of patients in whom blood cultures were obtained. The goal is to improve quality by early determination of the etiology of CAP.

EVALUATION OF VARIANCE FROM RECOMMENDED CARE

Result of sputum Gram stain and culture may not be available in less than 72 hours in patients who are unable to produce a sputum sample. This clinical situation is considered a justified variance. It is rare to have a justified medical reason not to obtain blood cultures in all hospitalized patients with CAP. A common clinical scenario that justifies the collection of blood cultures with the patient already on antibiotic therapy is the patient with CAP who is hospitalized owing to failure of outpatient antibiotic therapy.

REFERENCES

1. Niederman MS, Mandell LA, Anzueto A, et al: Guidelines for the management of adults with community-acquired pneumonia. American Thoracic Society. *Am J Respir Crit Care Med* 2001;163:1730–1754.
2. Bartlett JG, Dowell SF, Mandell LA, et al: Practice guidelines for the management of community-acquired pneumonia in adults. Guidelines from the Infectious Diseases Society of America. *Clin Infect Dis* 2000;31:347–382.

6
Empiric Antimicrobial Therapy

Classification of Patients
Patients Hospitalized in the General Medical Ward
Patients Hospitalized in the General Ward without Risk Factors for Resistant Organisms • Patients Hospitalized in the General Ward with Risk Factors for Resistant Organisms
Patients Hospitalized in the Intensive Care Unit
Patients Hospitalized in the Intensive Care Unit without Risk Factors for *Pseudomonas* • Patients Hospitalized in the Intensive Care Unit with Risk Factors for *Pseudomonas*
Timing of Antibiotic Administration
Evaluation of Local Practice
Quality Indicators
Proportion of Patients Admitted to the General Ward Treated with Appropriate Empiric Therapy • Proportion of Patients Admitted to the Intensive Care Unit Treated with Appropriate Empiric Therapy • Proportion of Patients with Empiric Therapy Given within 8 Hours of Arrival at the Hospital • Proportion of Patients with Empiric Therapy Given within 8 Hours of Diagnosis of Community-Acquired Pneumonia
Evaluation of Variance from Recommended Care
References

CLASSIFICATION OF PATIENTS

The American Thoracic Society (ATS) and the Infectious Diseases Society of America (IDSA) have proposed very similar guidelines for the selection of empiric antimicrobial therapy of hospitalized patients with community-acquired pneumonia (CAP).[1,2] Patients are initially classified in two groups according to severity of disease and site of care in the hospital. One group is composed of patients with moderate pneumonia who are hospitalized in the general medical ward; and the other includes patients with severe pneumonia who are hospitalized in intensive care units (ICUs).

PATIENTS HOSPITALIZED IN THE GENERAL MEDICAL WARD

According to the ATS guidelines, patients admitted to a general ward can be classified in two groups based on the presence of risk factors for penicillin-resistant *Streptococcus pneumoniae* and enteric gram-negative rods. Those considered at risk of infection with penicillin-resistant organisms include the elderly, patients with multiple medical comorbidities, patients with recent use of betalactam antibiotics, patients who are immunosuppressed, or patients in contact with a child in day care. The same factors are considered to place a patient at risk for infection with macrolide-resistant *S. pneumoniae*. Risk factors for the presence of enteric

TABLE 1. *Empiric therapy for patients hospitalized in a ward without risk factors for resistant organisms*

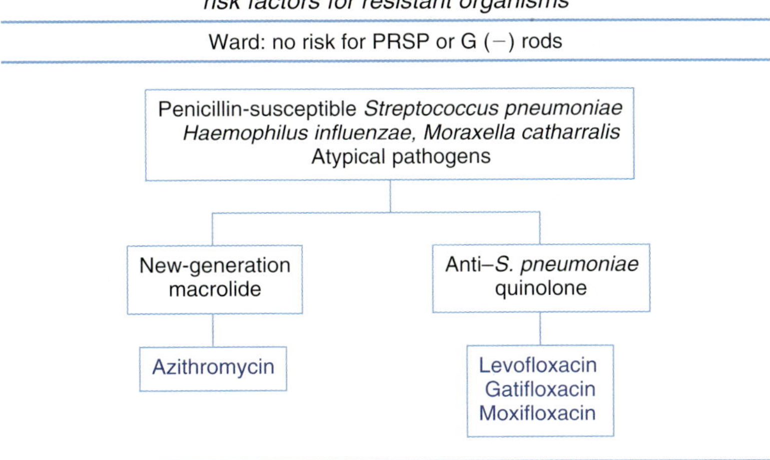

G (−), gram-negative; PRSP, penicillin-resistant *Streptococcus pneumoniae.*

Gram-negative organisms include the recent use of broad-spectrum antibiotics, the use of high-dose steroids, multiple medical comorbidities, and recent hospitalization.

Patients Hospitalized in the General Ward without Risk Factors for Resistant Organisms

Two types of regimens can be considered appropriate for initial empiric therapy for the hospitalized patient in the general ward without risk factors for the presence of resistant organisms. One regimen consists of monotherapy with a new-generation macrolide antibiotic; the other regimen consists of monotherapy with an anti-streptococcal quinolone. The most common organisms causing CAP in this group of patients and the most commonly used antibiotics for empiric therapy are presented in Table 1.

Patients Hospitalized in the General Ward with Risk Factors for Resistant Organisms

Two types of regimens can be considered appropriate for initial empiric therapy for the hospitalized patient in the general ward with risk factors for the presence of resistant organisms. One regimen consists of combination therapy with a betalactam antibiotic with good activity against resistant *S. pneumoniae* plus a macrolide antibiotic; the other regimen consists of monotherapy with an anti-streptococcal quinolone. The most common organisms causing CAP in this group of patients and the most commonly used antibiotics for empiric therapy are presented in Table 2.

PATIENTS HOSPITALIZED IN THE INTENSIVE CARE UNIT

Patients admitted to intensive care should be subclassified in two groups according to the presence of risk factors for *Pseudomonas aeruginosa* infection. Patients with chronic ob-

TABLE 2. *Empiric therapy for patients hospitalized in a ward with risk factors for resistant organisms*

Ward: risk for PRSP or G (−) rods

Penicillin-resistant *Streptococcus pneumoniae*
Haemophilus influenzae, Moraxella catharralis
Atypical pathogens, Enterobacteriaceae

- Beta-lactam plus Macrolide
  - Cefotaxime, Ceftriaxone
  - Erythromycin, Azithromycin
- Anti–*S. pneumoniae* quinolone
  - Levofloxacin, Gatifloxacin, Moxifloxacin

G (−), gram-negative; PRSP, penicillin-resistant *Streptococcus pneumoniae.*

structive pulmonary disease (COPD) complicated with bronchiectasis or patients with COPD and chronic use of broad-spectrum antibiotics can be colonized with gram-negative rods, including *P. aeruginosa*. When these patients are hospitalized to the ICU with severe CAP, they should be considered at risk for *P. aeruginosa* infection.

Patients Hospitalized in the Intensive Care Unit without Risk Factors for *Pseudomonas*

Two types of regimens can be considered appropriate empiric therapy for patients without risk factors for *Pseudomonas* infection. One regimen consists of a combination of betalactam antibiotic plus a macrolide; the other consists of a combination of betalactam antibiotic plus an anti-streptococcal quinolone. The betalactam antibiotic should have good activity against resistant pneumococci. Selecting a betalactam antibiotic with good activity against *P. aeruginosa* in this group of patients is not necessary. The lack of recommendation in national guidelines for the use of empiric therapy with a quinolone as monotherapy in this group of patients is due to a lack of clinical studies in patients with severe CAP admitted to the ICU. The most commonly used antibiotics recommended for each regimen are presented in Table 3.

Patients Hospitalized in the Intensive Care Unit with Risk Factors for *Pseudomonas*

Three types of regimens can be considered appropriate therapy for patients with risk factors for *Pseudomonas* infection. All regimens include an antipseudomonal betalactam antibiotic that can be combined with an antipseudomonal quinolone, or a macrolide, or an antistreptococcal quinolone. The selected betalactam should have activity against *P. aeruginosa* and should maintain activity against resistant pneumococci. The most commonly used antibiotics recommended for each regimen are presented in Table 4. The addition of single daily dose aminoglycoside is sometimes recommended until the presence of *P. aeruginosa* pneumonia with bacteremia has been ruled out.

TABLE 3. *Empiric therapy for patients hospitalized in an intensive care unit with no risk factors for* Pseudomonas aeruginosa *infection*

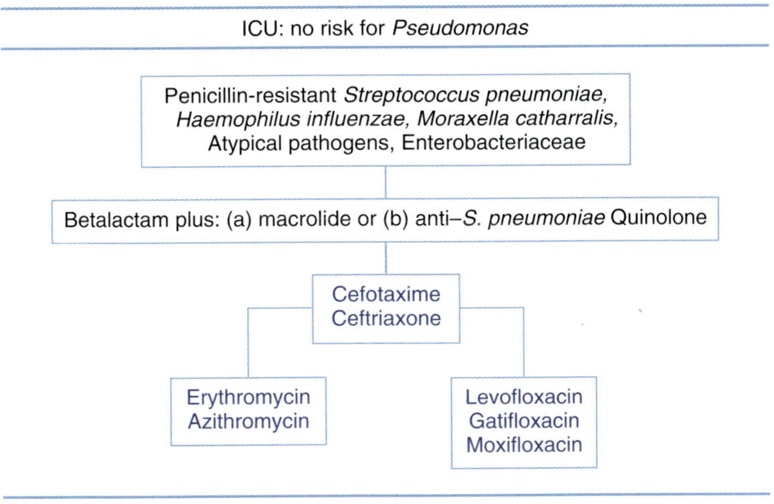

ICU, intensive care unit.

TIMING OF ANTIBIOTIC ADMINISTRATION

Recent data in the management of CAP indicate that delay in the initiation of anti-infective therapy is associated with longer hospital stay and decreased patient outcome.[3] Thus, it is suggested that hospitalized patients with CAP should have prompt initiation of empiric therapy.

A delay in administration of antibiotic may be secondary to a delay from a patient waiting to be seen by a physician after the patient arrived at the emergency room or a delay in the administration of antibiotics after the diagnosis of CAP was already performed.

TABLE 4. *Empiric therapy for patients hospitalized in an intensive care unit with risk factors for* Pseudomonas aeruginosa *infection*

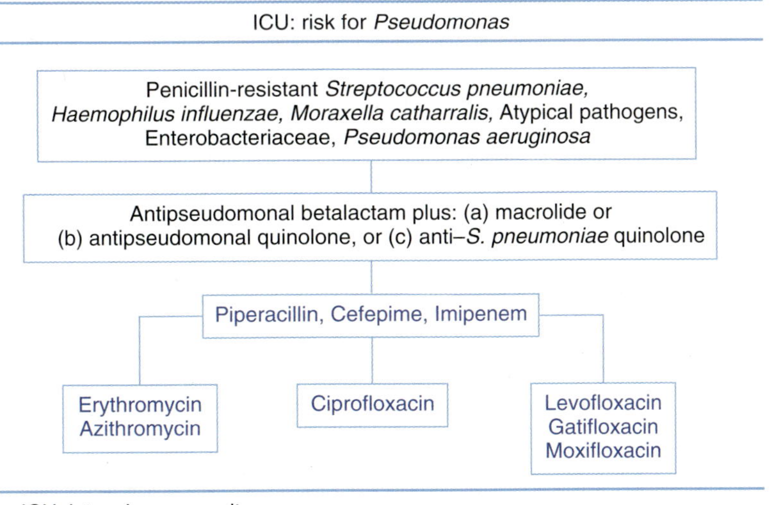

ICU, intensive care unit.

EVALUATION OF LOCAL PRACTICE

The initial empiric therapy can be selected as an area for evaluation of local practice. In our institution, patients meet guideline criteria for appropriate empiric therapy when the antibiotic selection is in compliance with the ATS or IDSA guidelines and the first antibiotic dose is given within 8 hours of patient arrival at the hospital. A sample form to collect data on quality indicators for the evaluation of this area of practice can be found in the Appendix. A current update of the literature in this area of practice can be found at www.caposite.com.

QUALITY INDICATORS

Proportion of Patients Admitted to the General Ward Treated with Appropriate Empiric Therapy

The proportion of patients admitted to a general ward who are treated with appropriate empiric therapy can be used as a quality indicator. For this indicator, the numerator is the number of patients admitted to the ward who were treated with appropriate empiric therapy, and the denominator is the total number of patients with CAP admitted to the ward. The goal is to improve patient clinical outcome by using appropriate initial empiric therapy.

Proportion of Patients Admitted to the Intensive Care Unit Treated with Appropriate Empiric Therapy

The proportion of patients admitted to ICU who are treated with appropriate empiric therapy can be used as a quality indicator. For this indicator, the numerator is the number of patients admitted to the ICU who were treated with appropriate empiric therapy, and the denominator is the total number of patients with the diagnosis of CAP admitted to the ICU. The goal is to improve patient clinical outcome by using appropriate initial empiric therapy.

Proportion of Patients with Empiric Therapy Given within 8 Hours of Arrival at the Hospital

The proportion of patients in whom empiric therapy was initiated within 8 hours of arrival can be used as a quality indicator. For this indicator, the numerator is the number of hospitalized patients with empiric therapy initiated within 8 hours of arrival, and the denominator is the total number of hospitalized patients with the diagnosis of CAP. The goal is to improve clinical outcome and decrease length of hospitalization by early initiation of empiric therapy.

Proportion of Patients with Empiric Therapy Given within 8 Hours of Diagnosis of CAP

The proportion of patients in whom empiric therapy was initiated within 8 hours of diagnosis of CAP can be used as a quality indicator. For this indicator, the numerator is the number of hospitalized patients with empiric therapy initiated within 8 hours of diagnosis, and the denominator is the total number of hospitalized patients with the diagnosis of CAP. The goal is to improve clinical outcome and decrease length of hospitalization by early initiation of empiric therapy.

EVALUATION OF VARIANCE FROM RECOMMENDED CARE

The initial empiric therapy suggested in all guidelines for hospitalized patients with CAP is designed for patients without acquired immunodeficiency syndrome (AIDS) or any other condition associated with immunosuppression. Because CAP in the immunocompromised patient can be produced by opportunistic pathogens, the initial empiric therapy suggested in a clinical guideline may not be appropriate for these patients. In the clinical situation in which the patient is at risk for unusual organisms, a variance from the antibiotic suggested in the guidelines is considered a justified variance. A common scenario is a patient with AIDS admitted to the hospital with CAP in whom trimethoprim/sulfamethoxazole is used as part of initial empiric therapy. Although the use of trimethoprim/sulfamethoxazole is not recommneded as empiric therapy in national guidelines, the deviation from recommendations in this patient is clinically justified.

It is unlikely to have a justified reason for a delay of more than 8 hours in antibiotic administration after a patient arrived at the hospital or after a patient was diagnosed with CAP.

REFERENCES

1. Niederman MS, Mandell LA, Anzueto A, et al:. Guidelines for the management of adults with community-acquired pneumonia. American Thoracic Society. *Am J Respir Crit Care Med* 2001;163:1730–1754.
2. Bartlett JG, Dowell SF, Mandell LA, et al: Practice guidelines for the management of community-acquired pneumonia in adults. Guidelines from the Infectious Diseases Society of America. *Clin Infect Dis* 2000;31:347–382.
3. Meehan TP, Fine MJ, Krumholz HM, et al: Quality of care, process and outcomes in elderly patients with pneumonia. *JAMA* 1997;278:2080–2084.

7

Switch from Intravenous to Oral Therapy

Pneumonia Recovery Phase
Switch Therapy
Switch Therapy Criteria
Oral Antimicrobial Therapy
Evaluation of Local Practice
Quality Indicator
Proportion of Patients with Appropriate Switch Therapy Performed
Evaluation of Variance from Recommended Care
References

PNEUMONIA RECOVERY PHASE

After initiation of intravenous empiric therapy, the majority of hospitalized patients will enter a recovery phase that will end with the clinical cure of the patient and the eradication of the pathogen. The recovery phase of hospitalized patients with community-acquired pneumonia (CAP) can be divided into three different periods (Fig. 1).[1] The first period starts with the initiation of antimicrobial therapy. During this first period, the patient is clinically unstable. The initial antimicrobial regimen should not be changed within this first period, unless there is a marked clinical deterioration. Even with appropriate empiric antimicrobial therapy, the majority of patients will remain clinically unstable for 48 to 72 hours. This first period ends when the patient reaches the point of clinical stability. During the second period, the patient shows evidence of initial clinical improvement. The signs, symptoms, and laboratory abnormalities caused by the infection begin to normalize. This second period of initial clinical improvement may last 24 to 48 hours. The third period is characterized by a definitive clinical improvement. During this period of recovery, the signs, symptoms, and laboratory abnormalities are greatly improved. This period occurs in the majority of patients after 5 days of hospitalization. This last period ends at the point of complete resolution of signs and symptoms, when the patient is considered clinically cured. National guidelines from the American Thoracic Society (ATS) and Infectious Diseases Society (IDSA) suggest that in patients who are clinically improving, the initial intravenous therapy can be switched to oral therapy (switch therapy).[2,3]

SWITCH THERAPY

The traditional approach to therapy of hospitalized patients with CAP has been the use of intravenous antibiotics during the entire recovery phase until the patient achieved definitive

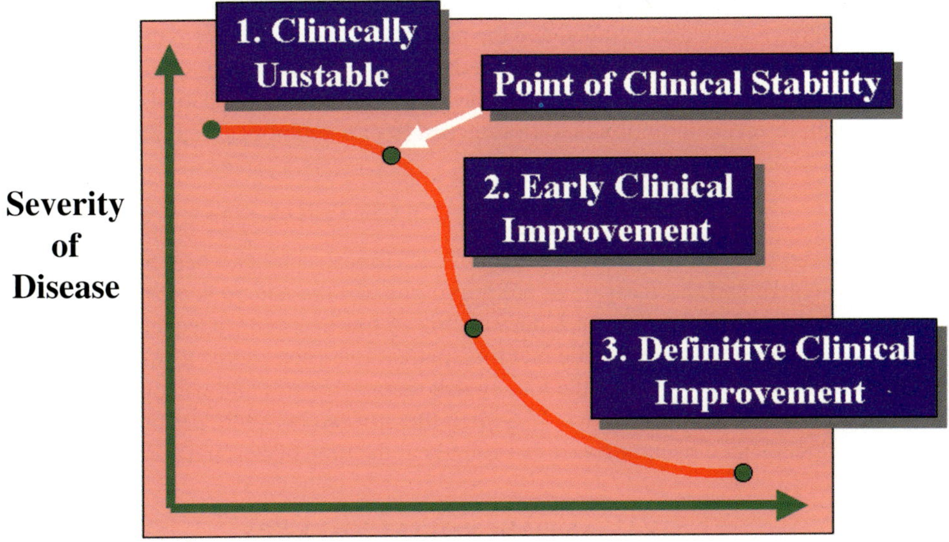

FIG. 1. The three periods during the recovery phase of hospitalized patients with community-acquired pneumonia. (From Ramirez JA: Switch therapy in adult patients with pneumonia. Clin Pulm Med 1995; 2[6]:327–333, with permission.)

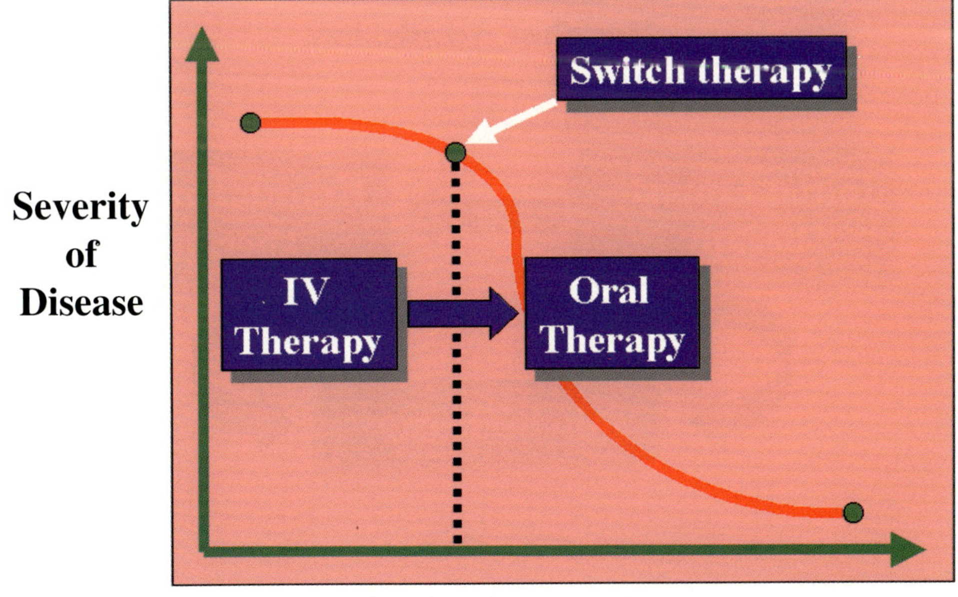

FIG. 2. The switch from intravenous (IV) to oral antibiotics is performed at the point of clinical stability.

clinical improvement. At this point, usually after several days of hospitalization, the intravenous antibiotics were discontinued and the patient was discharged from the hospital.

With the switch therapy approach, one needs to identify the point of clinical stability during the recovery phase. At this point, when the patient is entering the period of initial clinical improvement, intravenous antibiotics are switched to oral antibiotics (Fig. 2).

SWITCH THERAPY CRITERIA

A patient can be considered to reach the point of clinical stability when these three criteria are met: (a) cough and shortness of air are improving, (b) the patient is afebrile for at least 8 hours, (c) the white blood cell count is normalizing. A fourth criteria, adequate oral intake and gastrointestinal absorption, should be met for a patient to be considered a switch therapy candidate. As soon as a patient meets the four switch therapy criteria, intravenous antibiotics can be safely switched to oral antibiotics.[4,5] Switch therapy can be safely performed even in patients with documented pneumococcal bacteremia at the time of hospital admission[6]

ORAL ANTIMICROBIAL THERAPY

In hospitalized patients with CAP, the etiologic agent remains unknown in more than half of the cases. Because of this, the most common scenario in the management of CAP is a switch to oral antibiotics from empiric parenteral therapy (Fig. 3).

In this clinical situation, the oral antimicrobial should be equivalent to the intravenous empiric regimen with regard to spectrum of antimicrobial activity. If more than one oral antimicrobial is able to match the microbiologic activity of the intravenous regimen, the drug with

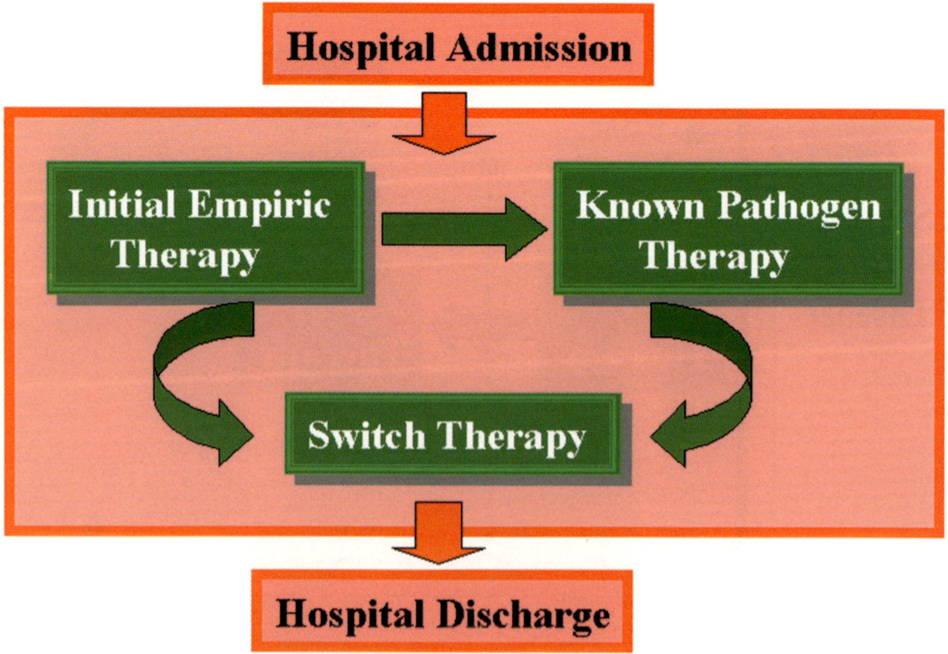

FIG. 3. Switch therapy can be performed in a patient with community-acquired pneumonia with a known or an unknown etiology.

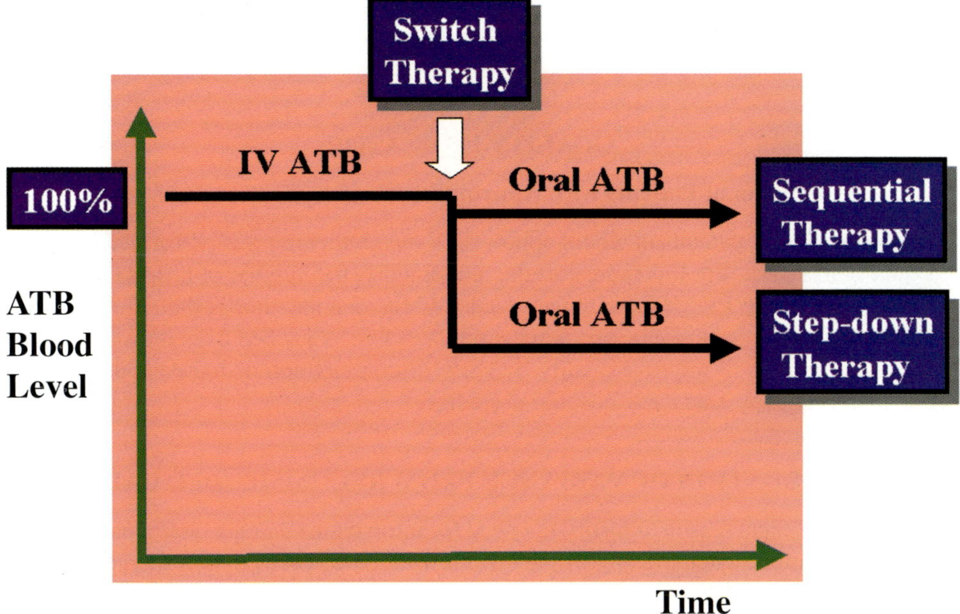

FIG. 4. Representation of sequential therapy and step-down therapy according to blood level achieved after switch therapy.ATB, antibiotic; IV, intravenous.

the best pharmacokinetic profile is selected. In patients with a known pathogen, the choice of the oral antimicrobial for switch therapy is based on the susceptibility pattern of the identified microorganism. In this clinical situation, the switch to oral antimicrobials is made from known pathogen therapy. If more than one oral antimicrobial is active against the etiologic agent, the antimicrobial with the narrowest spectrum of activity and best pharmacokinetic profile is chosen. Considering the antibiotic blood level achieved with the oral antibiotic in relation to that of the intravenous antibiotic, the switch to oral therapy can be defined as sequential therapy or step-down therapy (Fig. 4).

If the oral antibiotic achieved almost the same level as the intravenous formulation, the switch can be defined as sequential therapy (e.g., switch to oral quinolone antibiotic). If the oral antibiotic achieved a lower concentration than the intravenous formulation, the switch can be defined as step-down therapy (e.g., switch to oral macrolide or cephalosporin antibiotic). Good clinical outcome has been demonstrated with switch therapy using the sequential or step-down approach.

EVALUATION OF LOCAL PRACTICE

Switch therapy can be selected as an area for evaluation of local practice. In our institution, patients meet guideline criteria for appropriate switch therapy when they are switched to an appropriate oral antibiotic during the 24-hour period after the patient is a switch therapy candidate. A patient is considered a switch therapy candidate the day these four criteria are met: (a) cough and shortness of air are improving, (b) the patient is afebrile for at least 8 hours, (c) the white blood cell count is normalizing, and (d) the patient has adequate oral intake and gastrointestinal absorption. There is no need for continuation of intravenous therapy once the patient is a switch therapy candidate. A sample form to collect data on quality indicators for the evaluation of this area of practice can be found in the Appendix. A current update of the literature in this area of practice can be found at www.caposite.com.

QUALITY INDICATOR

Proportion of Patients with Appropriate Switch Therapy Performed

The proportion of patients in whom appropriate switch therapy was performed can be used as a quality indicator. For this indicator, the numerator is the number of hospitalized patients in whom appropriate switch therapy was used, and the denominator is the number of hospitalized patients with pneumonia who were candidates to be switched from intravenous to oral therapy. The goal is to improve quality by early discontinuation of intravenous lines, early switch to oral therapy, and early hospital discharge.

EVALUATION OF VARIANCE FROM RECOMMENDED CARE

There is no clinical reason to justify the need for intravenous therapy once a patient has met the four criteria for switch therapy. If the switch from intravenous to oral therapy is delayed more than 24 hours after a patient meets switch therapy criteria, the variance from recommended care is considered unjustified.

REFERENCES

1. Ramirez JA: Switch therapy in adult patients with pneumonia. *Clin Pulm Med* 1995;2:327–333.
2. Niederman MS, Mandell LA, Anzueto A, et al: Guidelines for the management of adults with community-acquired pneumonia. American Thoracic Society. *Am J Respir Crit Care Med* 2001;163:1730–1754.
3. Bartlett JG, Dowell SF, Mandell LA, et al:. Practice guidelines for the management of community-acquired pneumonia in adults. Guidelines from the Infectious Diseases Society of America. *Clin Infect Dis* 2000;31:347–382.
4. Ramirez JA, Srinath L, Ahkee S, et al: Early switch from intravenous to oral cephalosporins in the treatment of hospitalized patients with community-acquired pneumonia. *Arch Intern Med.* 1995;155:1273–1276.
5. Ramirez JA, Vargas S, Ritter GW, et al: Early switch from intravenous to oral antibiotics and early hospital discharge. *Arch Intern Med* 1999;159:2449–2454.
6. Ramirez JA, Bordon J: Early switch from intravenous to oral antibiotics in hospitalized patients with bacteremic *Streptococcus pneumoniae* community-acquired pneumonia. *Arch Intern Med* 2001;161:848–850.

8
Hospital Discharge

Clinical Response
Length of Stay Related Only to Community-Acquired Pneumonia
Length of Stay Related Not Only to Community-Acquired Pneumonia
Hospital Discharge Criteria
Resource Utilization
Evaluation of Local Practice
Quality Indicator
Proportion of Patients with Appropriate Length of Hospital Stay
Evaluation of Variance from Recommended Care
References

CLINICAL RESPONSE

A documented good clinical response to antibiotic therapy is one of the primary criteria in considering a patient ready for hospital discharge. The same criteria used to define when a patient is a candidate for switch therapy can be used to document a good clinical response.

From the group of hospitalized patients with good clinical response, some patients are candidates for hospital discharge the same day they are candidates for switch therapy, but a group of patients may need to continue in the hospital owing to other justified reasons even after they are switched to oral therapy.

LENGTH OF STAY RELATED ONLY TO COMMUNITY-ACQUIRED PNEUMONIA

The most common scenario for hospitalized patients with community-acquired pneumonia (CAP) is a rapid clinical improvement after initiation of appropriate empiric therapy. The great majority of these patients can be switched to oral therapy and discharged from the hospital to complete the course of therapy at home.[1] Once a patient is switched to oral therapy, there is no need to maintain the patient in the hospital for a period of observation to evaluate the clinical response to oral therapy.[2]

Because length of hospitalization is not influenced by any other factor outside of the pulmonary infection, patients are considered to have length of stay related only to pneumonia. In this type of patient, the length of hospital stay can be considered inappropriate if the switch to oral antibiotic was delayed more than 24 hours after the patient was considered a candidate for switch therapy or if the patient remains hospitalized for clinical observation in oral therapy.

LENGTH OF STAY RELATED NOT ONLY TO COMMUNITY-ACQUIRED PNEUMONIA

Some hospitalized patients will improve clinically and may be switched from intravenous to oral therapy but will need to remain hospitalized for other reasons.[1] Considering the possible clinical scenarios, these types of patients can be classified in three groups.

Group 1: Treatment of comorbidity. This group consists of patients who require medical treatment of a previous or new medical condition that worsened as a consequence of the pulmonary infection. No need for treatment of comorbid conditions is a well-established criteria for hospital discharge.[3] An example of deterioration of a previous medical condition is a patient with a well-known history of diabetes who developed severe metabolic abnormalities as a consequence of the pulmonary infection and may require hospital care even after the switch to oral therapy. An example of a new medical condition is a patient with a history of coronary artery disease who developed a new myocardial infarction after hospitalization. The patient may have a good clinical response of the pulmonary infection but needs to remain in the hospital for management of the myocardial infarction.

Group 2: Diagnostic workup. This group consists of patients in whom it is necessary to perform a diagnostic workup of a new medical condition that developed during the treatment of pulmonary infection. Examples include a patient with CAP complicated with a new episode of gastrointestinal bleeding who may need to remain hospitalized for an endoscopic examination to define the etiology of the bleeding; or a patient with a new onset of cardiac arrhythmia who may require a diagnostic workup with a 24-hour Holter monitor.

Group 3: Social needs. This group consists of patients who, from the point of view of their medical problems, are clinically stable and ready to continue therapy outside of the hospital, but they have social needs that prevent hospital discharge. An example is an elderly patient with CAP who lives alone, without any help from family or friends, who may be required to remain in the hospital until appropriate social support can be obtained.

Patients in any of these three groups have a justified reason to remain hospitalized even after clinical improvement of pulmonary infection has been documented. In these patients, the length of hospital stay will not be considered related only to CAP but also to other medical or social conditions.

HOSPITAL DISCHARGE CRITERIA

Taking into account all these clinical scenarios, a patient can be considered a candidate for hospital discharge when these four criteria are met: (a) The patient is a candidate for switch therapy, (b) there is no need to treat comorbidity in the hospital setting, (c) there is no need for diagnostic workup in the hospital setting, and (d) the patient has no social needs. Patients should be discharged home on the day they meet these four criteria.[1]

RESOURCE UTILIZATION

The most important component of the daily medical care cost for hospitalized patients with CAP is the cost of the hospital bed, also referred to as hotel cost. It is estimated that in US hospitals, 59 percent of the median daily cost corresponds to the hotel cost and 41 percent to the nonroom costs.[4] Three levels of resource utilization can be described for all hospitalized patients with CAP, taking into account the time to clinical improvement and the time of hospital discharge. The first level of resource utilization extends from the time the patient is hospitalized until the patient reaches clinical stability. The primary resources utilized during this time are the hospital bed or hotel cost, the microbiologic workup to define etiology of CAP, the laboratory workup to define severity of CAP, and the initial intravenous antibiotics. The second level of resource utilization extends from the time the patient is switched to oral antibiotics until discharge home. The primary resources utilized during this time are the hospital bed and the treatment with oral antibiotics. The third level of resource utilization extends from the time the patient is discharged from the hospital until resolution of infection. The primary resources utilized during this period are the treatment with oral antibiotics and follow-up clinic visits.

Considering the previously described levels, three models of resource utilization (A, B, or C) can be described for the majority of hospitalized patients with CAP.

Model A. This model is illustrated by patients who reach clinical stability; are switched to oral therapy; and soon after are discharged from the hospital. The final outcome is clinical cure of CAP (Fig. 1).

Model B. This model is illustrated by patients who reach clinical stability; are switched to oral antibiotics; but for reasons other than the pulmonary infection need to remain hospitalized (Fig. 2). These patients have length of hospital stay owing not only to CAP but also to other medical or social conditions.

Model C. The third model is illustrated by patients without clinical improvement after initial empiric therapy. Approximately 10 percent to 20 percent of hospitalized patients with CAP suffer clinical deterioration even when empiric therapy is given in accordance with national guidelines. These patients continue in a high level of resource utilization owing to lack of clinical improvement (Fig. 3).

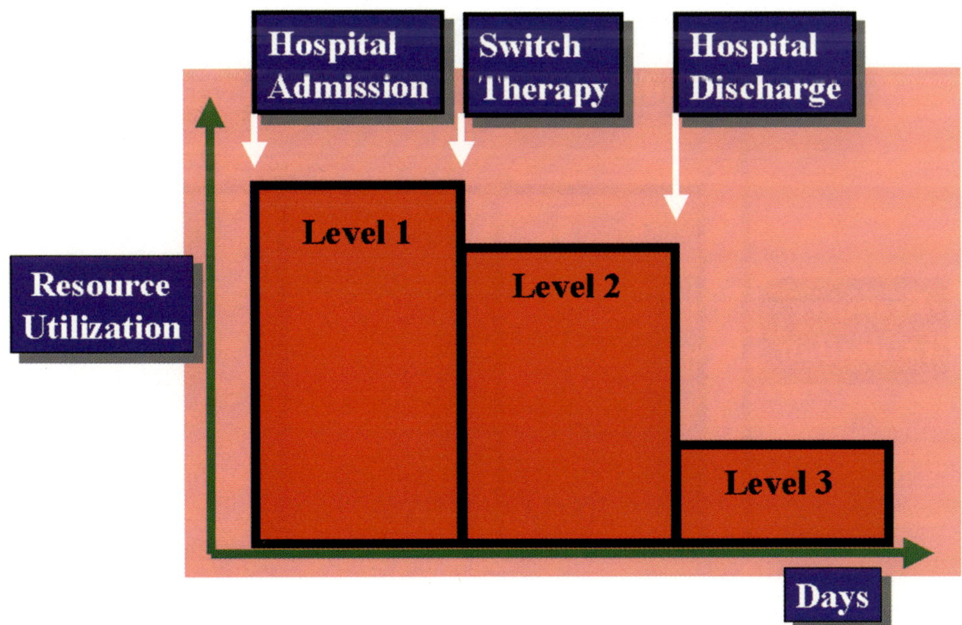

FIG. 1. Levels of resource utilization in a patient with switch therapy and length of stay related only to pneumonia (model A).

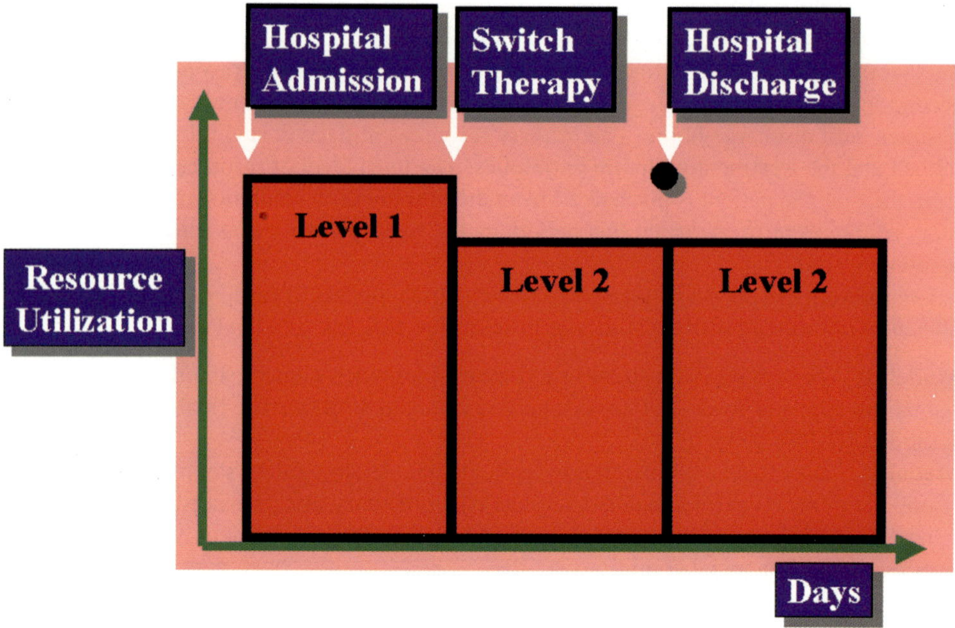

FIG. 2. Levels of resource utilization in a patient with switch therapy and length of stay related not only to pneumonia (model B).

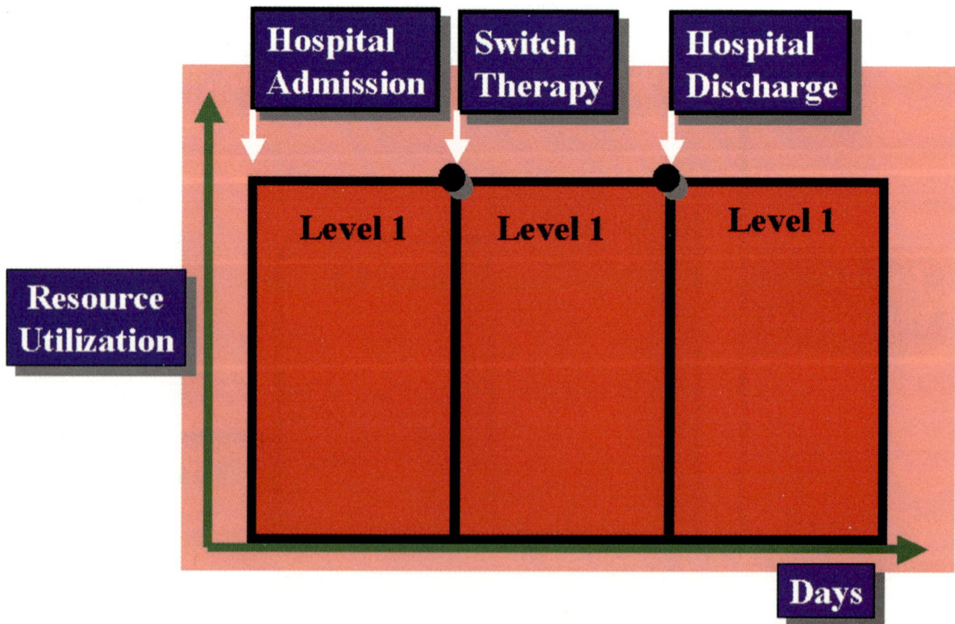

FIG. 3. Levels of resource utilization in a patient without clinical improvement (model C).

From the three described models of resource utilization, model A is the most cost-effective regarding clinical outcome and cost. In an attempt to apply this model to the great majority of hospitalized patients, the hospital CAP team needs to implement a program for optimal switch therapy and optimal hospital discharge.

EVALUATION OF LOCAL PRACTICE

The appropriateness of length of hospital stay can be selected as an area for evaluation of local practice. In our institution, patients meet guideline criteria for appropriate length of hospital stay when they are discharged from the hospital at the time these four criteria are met: (a) the patient is a candidate for switch therapy, (b) there is no need for further diagnostic workup in the hospital setting, (c) there is no need to treat comorbidity in the hospital setting, and (d) there are no unmet social needs. According to our hospital practice guideline, the length of hospital stay is considered appropriate if the patient is discharged from the hospital within 24 hours of becoming a candidate for hospital discharge. A sample form to collect data on quality indicators for the evaluation of this area of practice can be found in the Appendix. A current update of the literature in this area of practice can be found at www.caposite.com.

QUALITY INDICATOR

Proportion of Patients with Appropriate Length of Hospital Stay

The proportion of patients with appropriate length of hospital stay can be used as a quality indicator. For this indicator, the numerator is the number of hospitalized patients in whom appropriate length of hospital stay was documented, and the denominator is all hospitalized patients with CAP. The goal is to decreased cost of therapy by avoiding unnecessary hospital stay in patients who can be safely discharged home. Another important goal is to improve quality by preventing inappropriate hospital discharge in patients who will still benefit from hospital care.

EVALUATION OF VARIANCE FROM RECOMMENDED CARE

There is no clinical reason to justify the need for hospitalization once a patient has met the four criteria for hospital discharge. If the discharge is delayed more than 24 hours after a patient meets discharge criteria, the variance from recommended care is always considered unjustified.

REFERENCES

1. Ramirez JA, Vargas S, Ritter GW, et al: Early switch from intravenous to oral antibiotics and early hospital discharge. *Arch Intern Med* 1999;159:2449–2454.
2. Niederman MS, Mandell LA, Anzueto A, et al: Guidelines for the management of adults with community-acquired pneumonia. American Thoracic Society. *Am J Respir Crit Care Med* June. 2001;163:1730–1754.
3. Rhew DC, Tu GS, Ofman J, et al: Early switch and early discharge strategies in patients with community-acquired pneumonia. A meta-analysis. *Arch Intern Med* 2001;161:722–727.
4. Fine MJ, Pratt HM, Obrosky S, et al.: Relation between length of hospital stay and costs of care for patients with community-acquired pneumonia. *Am J Med* 2000;109:378–385.

9

Patient Education and Satisfaction with Care

Patient Education
Satisfaction with Care
Evaluation of Local Practice
Quality Indicators
Proportion of Patients with Education Performed • Proportion of Patients with Satisfaction with Care Evaluated • Proportion of Patients Who Were Not Sent Home Too Soon • Proportion of Patients Who Received Adequate Follow-up • Proportion of Patients Who Were Satisfied with the Care Received
Evaluation of Variance from Recommended Care
Reference

PATIENT EDUCATION

Education of the patient and/or the family regarding pneumonia should be an integral part of the management of the hospitalized patient with community-acquired pneumonia (CAP). Several objectives should be reached during the process of educating the patient. The patient should be able to understand what pneumonia is, what causes pneumonia, how pneumonia is treated, what type of support and treatment the patient will receive in the hospital, how soon recovery is expected, and how the patient can prevent a relapse, or a new episode of pneumonia. If the patient has any risk factor for tuberculosis (TB) and is placed on respiratory isolation, the patient should be educated and should understand what pulmonary TB is, why the patient is considered at risk for pulmonary TB, what the tuberculin test is, and why it is necessary for the patient to remain on respiratory isolation until the diagnosis of pulmonary TB has been ruled out.

In patients who are candidates to be switched from intravenous to oral antibiotics, education regarding the use of oral antimicrobials is of paramount importance. In this situation, the patient is discharged home with a partially treated infection, and appropriate use of antibiotics is critical to obtain adequate patient outcome. Before hospital discharge, the patient should be educated regarding the directions on how to use the oral antibiotics, importance of compliance, possible drug or food interaction, and side effects. The patient should have a good understanding of why the compliance with the oral antimicrobial is so important for the outcome.

Appropriate education of the patient and/or patient's family will have a favorable effect on patient outcome. A well-educated patient is more likely to be compliant with instructions during hospitalization, more likely to be compliant with oral antibiotics and other instructions after hospital discharge, and more likely to accept changes in lifestyle to prevent new episodes of pneumonia. From an institution perspective, patients who receive appropriate education during hospitalization will be more likely to be satisfied with the care they received.

SATISFACTION WITH CARE

The patients' judgments on certain aspects of the care of their infection determine their satisfaction or dissatisfaction with care. The patients' opinions about various aspects of care can be considered an outcome in relation to the management of pneumonia performed at a particular institution. In conjunction with patient clinical outcome, patient satisfaction with care is an important measurement to evaluate the quality of care received by the patient with CAP.

In our institution, we have a survey with these three questions to evaluate satisfaction with care:

1. Were you sent home too soon?
2. Did you receive adequate follow-up?
3. Are you satisfied with the care received?

EVALUATION OF LOCAL PRACTICE

Patient education and satisfaction with care can be selected as areas for evaluation of local practice. In our institution, practice guidelines for appropriate education were met when education was provided to a hospitalized patient with CAP. Guidelines for appropriate patient satisfaction with care were met when (a) patient satisfaction with care was documented, (b) the patient considered that he or she was not sent home too soon, (c) the patient considered that adequate follow-up was received, and (d) the patient was satisfied with the care received.

In institutions in which early switch to oral therapy and early hospital discharge are encouraged, patients are discharged home when they are still symptomatic. Our satisfaction with care indicates that 95 percent of the patients for whom the early switch and early discharge approach is used beleived the length of hospitalization was appropriate.[1] A sample to collect data on quality indicators for the evaluation of this area of practice can be found in the Appendix. A current update of the literature in this area of practice can be found at www.caposite.com.

QUALITY INDICATORS

Proportion of Patients with Education Performed

Data on the number of hospitalized patients and/or family who were educated about CAP can be used as a pneumonia quality indicator. For this indicator, the numerator is the number of hospitalized patients and/or family who were educated about CAP, and the denominator is the total number of hospitalized patients with CAP.

Proportion of Patients with Satisfaction with Care Evaluated

The proportion of patients with satisfaction with care evaluated can be used as a quality indicator. For this indicator, the numerator is the proportion of patients with known satisfaction with care, and the denominator is the total number of discharged patients with CAP.

Proportion of Patients Who Were Not Sent Home Too Soon

The proportion of patients who were not sent home too soon can be used as a quality indicator. For this indicator, the numerator is the number of patients considering the length of hospitalization to be adequate, and the denominator is the total number of patients with satisfaction with care evaluated.

Proportion of Patients Who Received Adequate Follow-up

The proportion of patients that received adequate follow-up can be used as a quality indicator. For this indicator the numerator is the total number of patients considering that they have received adequate follow-up, and the denominator is the total number of patients with satisfaction with care evaluated.

Proportion of Patients Who Were Satisfied with the Care Received

The proportion of patients who were satisfied with the care received can be used as a quality indicator. For this indicator, the numerator is the total number of patients considering that they have received adequate care, and the denominator is the total number of patients with satisfaction with care evaluated.

EVALUATION OF VARIANCE FROM RECOMMENDED CARE

Patient education regarding CAP may not be possible in hospitalized patients with deterioration of mental status. In this clinical scenario, variance from recommended patient education is considered justified. If data on patient satisfaction are collected by telephone survey, impossibility to contact the patient is a justified variance from recommended practice.

REFERENCE

1. Ramirez JA, Vargas S, Ritter GW, et al: Early switch from intravenous to oral antibiotics and early hospital discharge. *Arch Intern Med* 1999;159:2449–2454.

10
Clinical Outcome

Clinical Outcome
Clinical Course
Criteria for Clinical Improvement • Criteria for Clinical Deterioration • Classification of Clinical Deterioration
Evaluation of Local Practice
Quality Indicator
Proportion of Patients with Final Clinical Outcome Evaluated
Evaluation of Variance from Recommended Care
References

CLINICAL OUTCOME

The primary reason to develop and implement a practice guideline for the management of hospitalized patients with community-acquired pneumonia (CAP) is to improve patient outcome. Hospitals should have a system in place to evaluate clinical outcome in an attempt to document the number of patients with appropriate versus inappropriate outcome. With implementation of a local CAP practice guideline, it should be expected that the proportion of patients with outcome classified as clinical success will increase, and the proportion of patients classified as clinical failure will decrease.

During the clinical course of a patient with CAP, different times can be selected for evaluation of outcome. Clinical outcome can be evaluated at the time of hospital discharge. At this point, the patient with improvement of infection can be classified as clinical success, and the patient who died during hospitalization is classified as clinical failure. Evaluation of patient outcome at the time of hospital discharge is the simple way to evaluate and document clinical outcome. The problem with this form of evaluation is the inability to document a relapse of pneumonia or even death after discharge unless the patient is hospitalized in the same institution.

The ideal methodology to evaluate final clinical outcome is to examine all patients 3 to 4 weeks after therapy. At that point, a patient with resolution or improvement of infection is classified as clinical success, and a patient who died is classified as clinical failure. This outcome is sometimes difficult to capture owing to the need of a clinic visit for all patients. A follow-up telephone interview can simplify the evaluation of clinical outcome at 3 to 4 weeks after therapy.

The advantage of looking at final patient outcome is that outcome is evaluated at only one point in the clinical course of the disease, and the definitions used to classify a patient as clinical success or failure can be clearly delineated. One disadvantage of looking at outcome at the time of discharge or 3 to 4 weeks after therapy is that most of the resource utilization in hospitalized patients with CAP is related to the patient outcome during the first 7 days of hospi-

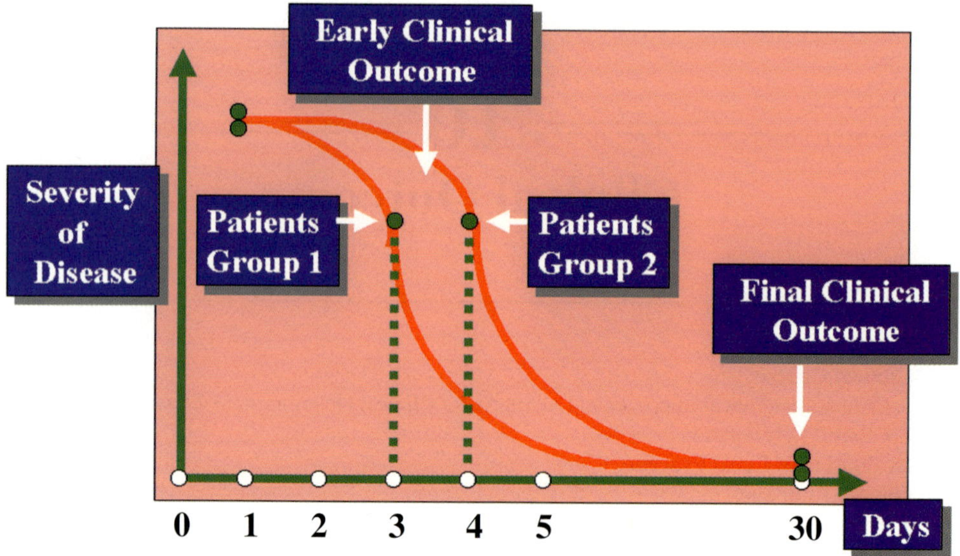

FIG. 1. Group of patients with equal final outcome but differences in time to clinical improvement and hospital discharge (early outcome).

talization. Theoretically, a group of patients who at 30 days have an equal clinical successful outcome may have a very different resource utilization if there is a significant difference in clinical outcome during the initial days of hospital therapy.

Figure 1 depicts an example of a series of patients treated with one antibiotic (group 1) who have the same clinical success at 30 days when compared with a group of patients treated with a different antibiotic (group 2). Although the clinical outcome at 30 days is equivalent, there is a significant difference among the groups regarding early clinical outcome. Because early clinical response is associated with early switch to oral therapy and early hospital discharge,

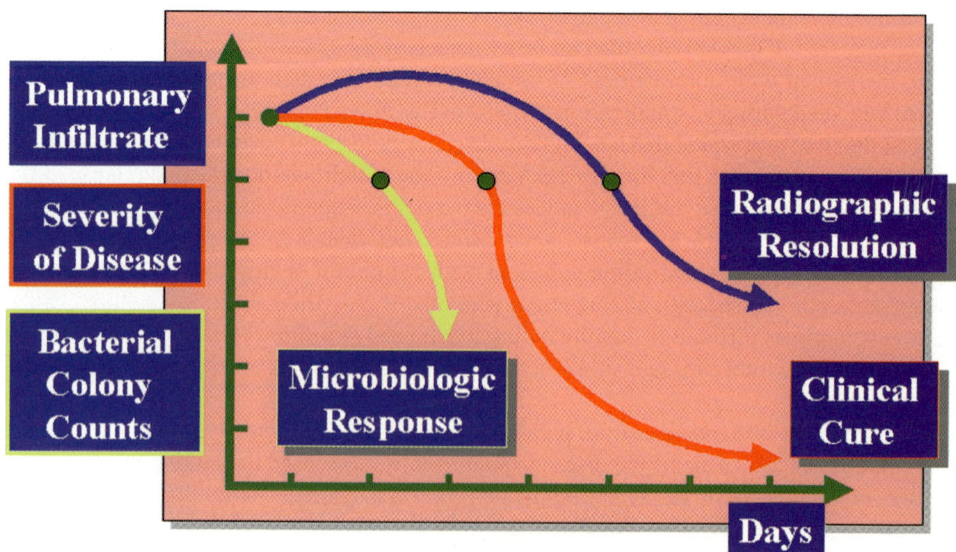

FIG. 2. Correlation of microbiologic response with clinical response and radiographic response in patients with community-acquired penumonia.

the resource utilization for group 1 is significantly less. If only final outcomes are to be evaluated, this important difference among groups will not be appreciated.

Early clinical outcomes are necessary to define the most cost-effective antimicrobial therapy. An antibiotic regimen that produces an earlier microbiologic resolution will be followed by an earlier clinical resolution. The correlation in the patterns of microbiologic response, clinical response, and radiographic response in patients with CAP is depicted in Figure 2.

If an institution is interested in evaluation of early clinical outcome, the clinical condition of the patient needs to be reviewed during the first days of hospitalization. To define early patient outcome, it is important to have a simple classification of the initial clinical course of hospitalized patients with CAP.

CLINICAL COURSE

After initiation of appropriate empiric therapy, the majority of hospitalized patients with CAP show evidence of clinical improvement by day 3 of treatment.[1,2] In some patients, the first evidence of clinical improvement may be delayed beyond 3 days owing to host or pathogen factors. In contrast to this frequent clinical course is a group of patients who, after initial antibiotic therapy, enter a phase of clinical deterioration. Clinical deterioration may occur early, during the first 3 days of therapy, or late, after 3 days of therapy. Some patients remain without significant changes in clinical status, without improvement or deterioration, beyond the first 7 days of hospitalization.

Based on this clinical response to therapy, the clinical outcome of patients with CAP may be categorized by day 7 of hospitalization into patients with early clinical response (group 1 of Fig. 3), patients with late clinical response (group 2 of Fig. 3), patients with early clinical deterioration (group 3 of Fig. 3), patients with late clinical deterioration (group 4 of Fig. 3), and patients with nonresolving CAP (group 5 of Fig. 3).

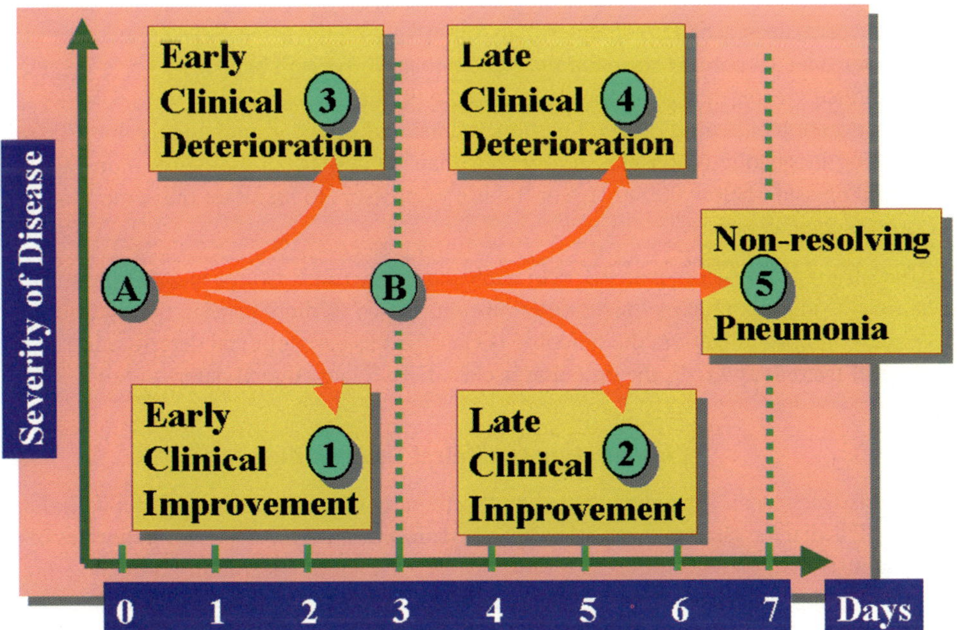

FIG. 3. Classification of the clinical course for patients with community-acquired pneumonia during the first 7 days of hospitalization.

Criteria for Clinical Improvement

In our institution, patients are considered to reach clinical improvement at the point they reach clinical stability and are candidates for switch therapy. Then, the clinical outcome is considered as clinical improvement when these three criteria are met: (a) cough and shortness of air are improving, (b) the patient is afebrile for at least 8 hours, and (c) the white blood cell count is normalizing. If criteria are met during the first 3 days of hospitalization, the outcome is classified as early clinical improvement. If criteria are met from days 4 to 7, the outcome is classified as late clinical improvement.

Criteria for Clinical Deterioration

Several parameters can be evaluated daily to assess response to therapy. The most commonly used are respiratory symptoms, fever, white blood cell count, pulmonary function, and hemodynamic function. Some patients develop a clear picture of clinical deterioration, requiring respiratory and hemodynamic support in a critical care unit. Then, the need for mechanical ventilation or transfer to an intensive care unit can be used as criteria to define clinical deterioration. Because a large number of patients who suffer clinical deterioration do not require mechanical ventilation or transfer to an intensive care unit, we have developed five criteria to define clinical deterioration based on the patient's symptoms, temperature, white blood cell count, pulmonary function, and hemodynamic function. The five criteria are

1. Deterioration of symptoms: manifested as increased cough, sputum, shortness of air, or pleuritic chest pain compared to the day before.
2. Deterioration of fever: manifested as an increase greater than 2° F from the previous day's maximal temperature.
3. Deterioration of the white blood cell count: manifested as an increase greater than 20 percent of leukocytes or greater than 50 percent in bands compared to the day before.
4. Deterioration of pulmonary function: manifested as increased respiratory rate greater than 50 percent, decreased Pa_{O_2} greater than 5 mmHg with the same F_{IO_2}, an increase in F_{IO_2} greater than 10 percent to maintain greater than 90 percent saturation, or a decrease in Pa_{O_2}/F_{IO_2} greater than 20 percent compared with the day before.
5. Deterioration of hemodynamic function: manifested as a heart rate greater than 20%, a reduction in systolic blood pressure greater than 40 mmHg, or a deterioration of systolic blood pressure below 90 mmHg, or the use of pressors to maintain the same blood pressure as the day before.

After hospital admission, patients who in the same day fulfill two or more of these five criteria are considered to have clinical deterioration. If two or more criteria are met during the first 3 days of hospitalization, the outcome is classified as early clinical deterioration. If criteria are met from days 4 to 7, the outcome is classified as late clinical deterioration.

Classification of Clinical Deterioration

One possible reason for failure to respond to therapy in hospitalized patients with diagnosis of CAP is that the clinical diagnosis of pneumonia was incorrect.[1,2] Some examples of clinical diagnosis that may be confused initially with CAP include obstructing bronchogenic carcinoma, lymphoma, intrapulmonary bleeding, bronchiolitis obliterans organizing pneumonia, and drug-induced pulmonary disease (e.g., amiodarone). A patient diagnosed with a noninfectious illness should be excluded from clinical outcome evaluation.

In patients with a correct diagnosis of CAP, the clinical deterioration can be classified in two groups, taking into consideration the antibiotic coverage of the initial empiric therapy: one group of patients with deterioration owing to inappropriate antimicrobial therapy, and a second group of patients with clinical deterioration even with appropriate antimicrobial therapy. Several etiologies can explain deterioration in each of the groups.

Clinical deterioration owing to inappropriate antimicrobial therapy

Even in patients with selection of antibiotic therapy in accordance to guidelines, the antibiotic may not cover the etiologic agent of CAP owing to the presence of an organism with unusual susceptibility (e.g., MRSA) or the presence of an unusual organism.[1,2] For some patients, an episode of CAP may be the first manifestation of an unrecognized immunodeficiency owing to human immunodeficiency virus (HIV) infection, malignancy, or other underlying disease, and the etiology of CAP may be an unusual organism that will not be appropriately covered with the standard empiric therapy recommended in the hospital guidelines (e.g., *Pneumocystis carinii* pneumonia [PCP] in a patient with unrecognized acquired immunodeficiency syndrome [AIDS]). In an attempt to identify an organism resistant to the initial antimicrobial therapy, all patients with clinical deterioration should have a more extensive microbiologic workup. The workup may include a pulmonary sample obtained by bronchoscopy with bronchoalveolar lavage.

Clinical deterioration with appropriate antimicrobial therapy

Clinical deterioration may occur in patients infected with common pathogens that are susceptible to the selected empiric antibiotics. For example, clinical deterioration may occur in a

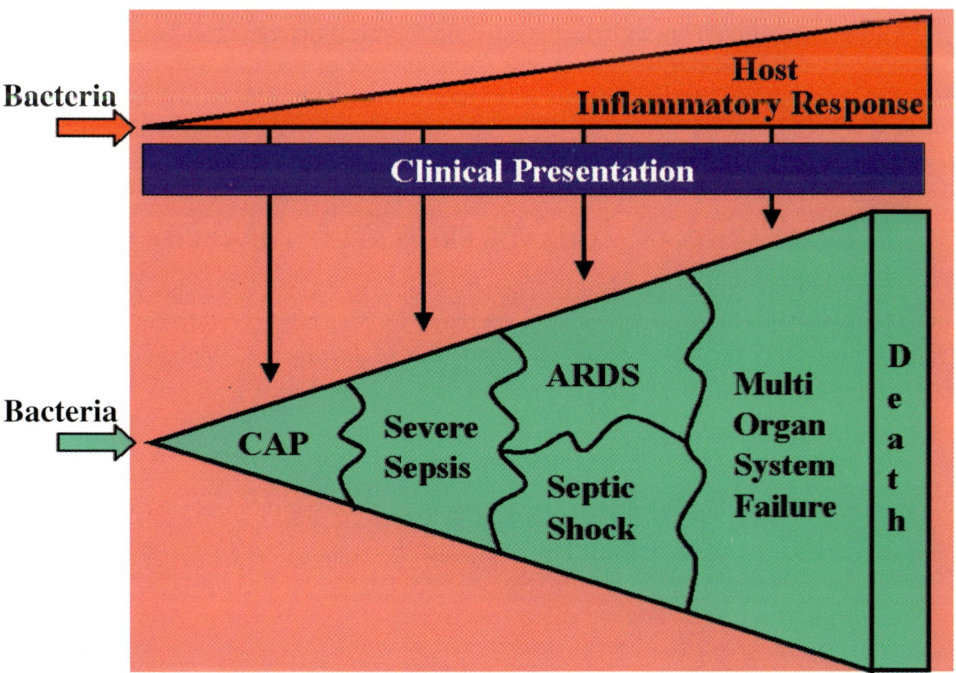

FIG. 4. Correlation of inflammatory response and clinical picture. CAP, community-acquired pneumonia; ARDS, acute respiratory distress syndrome.

patient infected with a susceptible *Streptococcus pneumoniae* who was started on appropriate empiric therapy. These are patients with severe pneumonia in whom the systemic inflammatory response to the pulmonary infection progresses even when they were started on appropriate therapy.[1,2] These patients admitted to the hospital with diagnosis of CAP will evolve into a clinical picture of severe sepsis, acute respiratory distress syndrome, septic shock, multiorgan failure, and death (Fig. 4).

The progression from CAP to severe sepsis ending with multiorgan failure due to an uncontrolled host inflammatory response is a common etiology of clinical deterioration in hospitalized patients with CAP.

Other causes of clinical deterioration in patients with appropriate antibiotic therapy of the pulmonary infection include a metastatic infection (e.g., empyema, pericarditis), a superimposed nosocomial infection (e.g., sinusitis, urinary tract infection), or a superimposed medical complication (e.g., pulmonary embolism, myocardial infarction).

EVALUATION OF LOCAL PRACTICE

The documentation of patient final outcome 3 to 5 weeks after hospitalization can be selected as an area for evaluation of local practice. In our institution, patients meet guideline criteria for appropriate evaluation of clinical outcome when there is documentation that indicates the patient's final clinical outcome. A sample form to collect data on quality indicators for the evaluation of this area of practice can be found in the Appendix. A current update of the literature in this area of practice can be found at www.caposite.com.

QUALITY INDICATOR

Proportion of Patients with Final Clinical Outcome Evaluated

The proportion of patients with documented final clinical outcome can be used as a quality indicator. For this indicator, the numerator is the number of patients with final clinical outcome documented, and the denominator is the total number of hospitalized patients with CAP. The goal is to improve quality by identification and evaluation of patients with poor outcome to identify areas of management that can be enhanced.

EVALUATION OF VARIANCE FROM RECOMMENDED CARE

Evaluation of final outcome requires a patient visit to a clinic or a telephone contact. In the clinical situation in which the patient does not return for a scheduled follow-up clinic visit and the patient cannot be contacted by telephone, the lack of documented final outcome is considered as a justified variance from recommended care.

REFERENCES

1. Niederman MS, Mandell LA, Anzueto A, et al: Guidelines for the management of adults with community-acquired pneumonia. American Thoracic Society. *Am J Respir Crit Care Med* 2001;163:1730–1754.
2. Bartlett JG, Dowell SF, Mandell LA, et al: Practice guidelines for the management of community-acquired pneumonia in adults. Guidelines from the Infectious Diseases Society of America. *Clin Infect Dis* 2000;31:347–382.

11
Pneumonia Prevention

Influenza and Pneumococcal Vaccines
Smoking Cessation
Evaluation of Local Practice
Quality Indicators
Proportion of Patients Evaluated for or Given Pneumococcal Vaccine • Proportion of Patients Evaluated for or Given Influenza Vaccine • Proportion of Patients with Smoking Cessation Offered
Evaluation of Variance from Recommended Care
References

INFLUENZA AND PNEUMOCOCCAL VACCINES

During epidemics of influenza, there is an increase in the frequency of community-acquired pneumonia (CAP) due to primary influenza pneumonia as well as secondary bacterial pneumonia complicating a case of influenza. Influenza vaccine is effective in limiting the severity of disease caused by the influenza virus. The pneumococcal vaccine has been proved to prevent pneumococcal pneumonia in young adults. The efficacy of the vaccine tends to decline with age and in patients who are immunocompromised.

The population of hospitalized patients with CAP should be consider a high-risk population for re-hospitalization related to influenza or pneumonia. All national guidelines consider that hospitalized patients with CAP should be evaluated to define whether they are candidates for vaccination, and candidates should be vaccinated before hospital discharge.[1,2]

There is no contraindication for the use of the pneumococcal vaccine and the influenza vaccine following an episode of CAP. These vaccines can be given simultaneously at different sites, without increasing side effects.[3]

When patients are hospitalized during the influenza season, they can be considered at risk of acquiring influenza from an infected health care worker. The vaccination of health care workers can be seen as an important strategy for the prevention of influenza in vulnerable hospitalized patients. Influenza vaccination of health care workers has been suggested as a pneumonia quality indicator.[4]

SMOKING CESSATION

Because smoking is a definitive risk factor for the acquisition of pneumonia, all hospitalized patients with CAP should be advised to be enrolled in a smoking cessation program in an attempt to prevent relapse of pneumonia. Members of the hospital CAP team should be aware of the recent pharmacological and behavioral therapies that have been used to assist smokers in overcoming their addiction.[5] Smoking cessation programs should be offered to all smokers.

EVALUATION OF LOCAL PRACTICE

The prevention of pneumonia can be selected as an area for evaluation of local practice. In our institution, patients meet guideline criteria for adequate prevention of CAP when: (1) they are evaluated prior to discharge from the hospital to see if whether they are candidates for influenza and/or pneumococcal vaccination, (2) patients identified as candidates received the vaccine prior to hospital discharge, and (3) patients that who smoke are offered an smoking cessation program. A sample of a form to collect data on quality indicators for the evaluation of this area of practice can be found in the Appendix. A current update of the literature in this area of practice can be found at www.caposite.com.

QUALITY INDICATORS

Proportion of Patients Evaluated for or Given Pneumococcal Vaccine

The proportion of patients evaluated for or given pneumococcal vaccine can be used as a quality indicator. For this indicator, the numerator is the total number of patients evaluated for or given pneumococcal vaccination, and the denominator is the total number of patients discharged with CAP. The goal is to improve quality by preventing a new episode of pneumococcal CAP.

Proportion of Patients Evaluated for or Given Influenza Vaccine

The proportion of patients evaluated for or given influenza vaccine can be used as a quality indicator. For this indicator, the numerator is the total number of patients that who were evaluated for of or given influenza vaccine, and the denominator is the total number of discharged patients with CAP during the influenza season. The goal is to improve quality by preventing influenza and its complications.

Proportion of Patients with Smoking Cessation Offered

The proportion of patients with smoking cessation offered can be used as a quality indicator. For this indicator, the numerator is the total number of patients to whom smoking cessation was offered, and the denominator is the total number of smoker patients who were discharged from the hospital with CAP. The goal is to improve quality by preventing new episodes of CAP.

EVALUATION OF VARIANCE FROM RECOMMENDED CARE

All hospitalized patients with CAP should be evaluated to see if they are candidates to receive the pneumococcal vaccine, and all candidates should be vaccinated. There is no justified medical reason for a variance from this indicator.

During the influenza season, all hospitalized patients with CAP should be evaluated to see if they are candidates to receive the influenza vaccine, and all candidates should be vaccinated. There is no justified medical reason for a variance from this indicator.

All smokers admitted to hospital with CAP should have a program for smoking cessation offered. There is no justified medical reason for a variance from this indicator.

REFERENCES

1. Niederman MS, Mandell LA, Anzueto A, et al: Guidelines for the management of adults with community-acquired pneumonia. American Thoracic Society. *Am J Respir Crit Care Med* 2001;163:1730–1754.
2. Bartlett JG, Dowell SF, Mandell LA, et al: Practice guidelines for the management of community-acquired pneumonia in adults. Guidelines from the Infectious Diseases Society of America. *Clin Infect Dis* 2000;31:347–382.
3. Fletcher TJ, Tunnicliffe WS, Hammond K, et al: Simultaneous immunization with influenza vaccine and pneumococcal polysaccharide vaccine in patients with chronic respiratory disease. *BMJ*,1997;314:1663–1665.
4. Rhew DC: Quality indicators for the management of pneumonia in vulnerable elders. *Ann Intern Med* 2001;135:736–743.
5. Rennard SI, Daughton DM: Smoking cessation. *Chest* 2000;117(5 Suppl 2):360S–364S.

Appendix

Sample form to collect data on quality indicators for evaluation of the management of hospitalized patients with community-acquired pneumonia (CAP). Eleven areas of practice with high impact on outcomes can be evaluated. For each quality indicator, the most common reasons for justified or unjustified variance from recommended care are depicted.

DIAGNOSIS OF COMMUNITY-ACQUIRED PNEUMONIA

Criteria for diagnosis of CAP*

A. X-ray with evidence of new pulmonary infiltrate (within 24 hours of admission) _____Yes _____No
B. New or increased cough with/without sputum production _____Yes _____No
C. Fever > 37.8°C (100.0° F) or hypothermia < 35.6°C (96.0°F) _____Yes _____No
D. Changes in white blood cell count (WBC) (leukocytosis, left shift, or leukopenia) _____Yes _____No

*Diagnosis of CAP requires the presence of criteria A (new pulmonary infiltrate) plus at least one of criteria B, C, and D.

Indicator: Did the patient meet the criteria for diagnosis of CAP?

_____ Yes, patient met criteria
_____ No, variance justified, pulmonary infiltrate evident 24 to 48 hours after admission
_____ No, variance justified, lack of infiltrate due to severe immunosuppression (e.g., acquired immunodeficiency syndrome [AIDS], neutropenia)
_____ No, variance justified, please comment
_____ No, variance unjustified, chronic pulmonary infiltrates
_____ No, variance unjustified, nosocomial pneumonia
_____ No, variance unjustified

Comment: ____

Indicator: Was CAP standard order form used?

_____ Yes, standard order form was used
_____ No, variance justified, patient admitted from clinic
_____ No, variance justified, transfer from another hospital
_____ No, variance justified, admitted with another diagnosis
_____ No, variance justified, admitted to intensive care unit (ICU)
_____ No, variance justified, please comment
_____ No, variance unjustified

Comment: ____

Need for Oxygen Therapy:

Indicator: Oxygenation assessment performed within 24 hours of diagnosis of pneumonia?

_____ Yes, select
    _____ Pulse oximetry
    _____ Arterial blood gases
    _____ Both pulse oximetry and arterial blood gases
_____ No, variance justified, please comment
_____ No,variance unjustified

Comment: ____

NEED FOR HOSPITALIZATION

To calculate the need for hospitalization, use the worst value at the time that decision for hospitalization was made.

A. Hospitalization Based on Risk Class

A. Is the patient older than 50 years? _____Yes _____No
B. Does the patient have any of the following coexisting conditions? _____Yes _____No
    Neoplastic disease (active or within the last year)
    Congestive heart failure
    Cerebrovascular disease
    Renal disease
    Liver disease
C. Does the patient have any of the following abnormalities on physical examination?
    ____Yes _____No
    Altered mental status
    Pulse ≥ 125/min
    Respiratory rate ≥ 30/min
    Systolic blood pressure < 90 mmHg
    Temperature < 35°C or ≥ 40°C (< 95°F or ≥ 104°F)

If answers to questions A, B, and C are all "No," the patient belongs to risk class I
If answer to A, B, or C is "Yes,"go to the following (check positive findings):

_____	1. Age [Men = (actual age)/Women = (age − 10 yr)]		
_____	2. Neoplastic disease	+30	_____ Risk class I
_____	3. Liver disease	+20	
_____	4. Congestive heart failure	+10	_____ Risk class II
_____	5. Cerebrovascular disease	+10	≤ 70 points
_____	6. Renal disease	+10	
_____	7. Altered mental status	+20	_____ Risk class III
_____	8. Respiratory rate ≥ 30/min	+20	71–90 points
_____	9. Systolic blood pressure < 90 mmHg	+20	
_____	10. Temperature < 35°C or ≥ 40°C (< 95.0°F or ≥ 104.0°F)	+15	_____ Risk Class IV
_____	11. Pulse ≥ 125/min	+10	91–130 points
_____	12. Nursing home resident	+10	

		Points	
_____	13. Arterial pH < 7.35	+30	_____ Risk class V
_____	14. Blood urea nitrogen (BUN) > 30 mg/dl	+20	> 130 points
_____	15. Sodium < 130 mmol/L	+20	
_____	16. Glucose ≥ 250 mg/dl	+10	
_____	17. Hematocrit < 30%	+10	
_____	18. $Po_2 < 60$ or $Po_2/FIo_2 < 300$ or O_2 Sat < 90%	+10	
_____	19. Pleural effusion	+10	

Total _____ **Assign to Risk Class**

Indicator: Did the patient meet criteria for hospitalization based on risk class? (Risk classes III, IV, V)

_____ Yes, patient is in risk class III, IV, or V
_____ No, variance justified, admitted owing to nausea/vomiting
_____ No, variance justified, admitted owing to noncompliance
_____ No, variance justified, admitted owing to social needs
_____ No, variance justified, admitted to rule out sepsis
_____ No, variance justified, admitted owing to failure of outpatient therapy
_____ No, variance justified, admitted owing to hypoxemia
_____ No, variance justified, admitted owing to other medical condition, please comment
_____ No, variance unjustified

Comment: ____

B. Hospitalization Based on Criteria for Complicated Course

Demographic Factors

_____ 1. Age > 65 years
_____ 2. Nursing home resident

Comorbid Illness

_____ 3. Chronic obstructive pulmonary disease (COPD)
_____ 4. Diabetes mellitus
_____ 5. Chronic renal failure
_____ 6. Congestive heart failure
_____ 7. Chronic liver disease (any etiology)
_____ 8. Prior admission for CAP within 1 year
_____ 9. Suspicion of aspiration
_____ 10. Neurologic diseases/mental illness
_____ 11. Post splenectomy state
_____ 12. Cerebrovascular disease
_____ 13. Neoplastic disease
_____ 14. Ethanol abuse/malnutrition
_____ 15. Other immunosuppressive state

Signs and Symptoms

_____ 16. Respiratory rate > 30/min
_____ 17. Diastolic blood pressure < 60 mmHg
_____ 18. Systolic blood pressure < 90mmHg
_____ 19. Pulse > 125/min
_____ 20. Temperature < 35.0°C (< 95.0°F)
_____ 21. Temperature ≥ 40.0°C (≥ 104.0°F)
_____ 22. Extrapulmonary site of infection
_____ 23. Altered mental status

Laboratory Findings

_____ 24. WBC < 4,000 or absolute neutrophil count (ANC) < 1,000
_____ 25. WBC > 20,000
_____ 26. Serum creatinine > 1.2 mg/dl
_____ 27. BUN > 30 mg/dl
_____ 28. Hematocrit<30% or hemoglobin < 9 g/dl
_____ 29. Albumin < 2.6 g/L
_____ 30. Platelet count < 100,000
_____ 31. Sodium < 130 mmol/L

____ 32. Glucose > 250 mg/dl
____ 33. P_{O_2} < 60 on room air or
Pa_{O_2}/F_{IO_2} < 300 or
O_2 Sat < 90%
____ 34. PCO_2 > 50 on room air
____ 35. Arterial pH< 7.35
____ 36. Need for mechanical ventilation
____ 37. Bacteremia

Chest X-ray Findings

____ 38. Multiple lobe involvement
____ 39. Presence of a cavity
____ 40. Pleural effusion

Following Etiology from Blood Cultures

____ 41. *Staphylococcus*
____ 42. Gram-negative rods

Number of risk factors for complicated course: ______

Indicator: Did the patient meet criteria for hospitalization based on risk for complicated course?
(> 1 risk factor)

_____ Yes, patient had more than one risk factor
_____ No, variance justified, admitted owing to nausea/vomiting
_____ No, variance justified, admitted owing to noncompliance
_____ No, variance justified, admitted owing to social needs
_____ No, variance justified, admitted to rule out sepsis
_____ No, variance justified, admitted owing to failure of outpatient therapy
_____ No, variance justified, admitted owing to hypoxemia
_____ No, variance justified, admitted owing to other medical condition, please comment
_____ No, variance unjustified

Comment: ____

NEED FOR RESPIRATORY ISOLATION

Risk Factors for Tuberculosis

Check all that apply:

Symptoms

_____ Night sweats _____ Hemoptysis _____ Weight loss _____ Hoarseness

Member of High-risk Group

_____ Human immunodeficiency virus (HIV)/AIDS-positive
_____ History of positive purified protein derivative (PPD)
_____ Homeless
_____ Alcohol/drug abuse
_____ Health care worker
_____ History of tuberculosis (TB)
_____ Age > 65 years
_____ Community living (prison, nursing home, shelter)
_____ Recent exposure to active TB
_____ From area with high risk of TB

History of Chronic Illness

_____ Silicosis
_____ End-stage renal disease
_____ Gastrectomy
_____ Cancer of mouth or gastrointestinal (GI) tract
_____ 10% or below ideal body weight
_____ Diabetes mellitus
_____ Hematologic disease
_____ Intestinal bypass
_____ Chronic malabsorption syndrome
_____ Long-term cortisone therapy
_____ Other immunosuppressive state ______________________________

Number of risk factors present: ______

Indicator: Was patient placed in respiratory isolation?

_____ Yes
_____ No, variance justified, did not meet criteria to be considered at risk for this institution
_____ No, variance justified, lack of isolation bed
_____ No, variance justified, please comment
_____ No, variance unjustified

Comment: ____

Indicator: Were acid-fact bacilli (AFB) smear and culture obtained within 24 hours of admission?

_____ Yes
_____ No, variance justified, no sputum production
_____ No, variance justified, not considered at risk
_____ No, variance justified, please comment
_____ No, variance unjustified

Comment: ____

Indicator: If patient was placed in isolation, were two AFB smears negative before isolation was discontinued?

_____ Yes
_____ No, variance justified, other etiology identified
_____ No, variance justified, please comment
_____ No, variance unjustified

Comment: ____

Indicator: If patient was placed in isolation, was isolation discontinued within 24 hours after two AFB smears were negative?

_____ Yes
_____ No, variance justified, please comment
_____ No, variance unjustified

Comment: ____

MICROBIOLOGIC WORKUP

Indicator: Sputum Gram stain results available ≤ 72 hours from admission?

_____ Yes
_____ No, variance justified, no sputum production
_____ No, variance justified, please comment
_____ No, variance unjustified, not ordered
_____ No, variance unjustified, sample not obtained
_____ No, variance unjustified, sample unacceptable
_____ No, variance unjustified, result available > 72 hours
_____ No, variance unjustified

Comment: ____

Indicator: Sputum culture results available ≤ 72 hours from admission?

_____ Yes
_____ No, variance justified, no sputum production
_____ No, variance justified, please comment
_____ No, variance unjustified, not ordered
_____ No, variance unjustified, sample not obtained
_____ No, variance unjustified, sample unacceptable
_____ No, variance unjustified, result available after 72 hours
_____ No, variance unjustified

Comment: ____

Indicator: Blood culture results available ≤ 72 hours from admission?

_____ Yes
_____ No, variance justified, please comment
_____ No, variance unjustified, culture not ordered
_____ No, variance unjustified, sample not obtained
_____ No, variance unjustified, result available after 72 hours
_____ No, variance unjustified

Comment: ____

Indicator: Were two sets of blood cultures obtained before antibiotics were given?

_____ Yes
_____ No, variance justified, please comment
_____ No, variance unjustified

Comment: ____

PATIENT EDUCATION

Indicator: Was patient education performed?

_____ Yes
_____ No, variance justified, patient unable to understand education
_____ No, variance justified, please comment
_____ No, variance unjustified

Comment: ____

EMPIRIC ANTIMICROBIAL THERAPY

- Patient arrival to hospital: Date _____ Time _____
- Positive x-ray indicating CAP: Date _____ Time _____
- Empiric therapy given: Date _____ Time _____

Antibiotics received as empiric therapy

Antimicrobial	Dose/Route/Frequency	Start Date	Stop Date

Indicator: Was empiric therapy in compliance with the local guidelines?

_____ Yes
_____ No, variance justified, risk for unusual organisms
_____ No, variance justified, please comment
_____ No, variance unjustified, excessive use
_____ No, variance unjustified, under use
_____ No, variance unjustified

Comment: ____

Indicator: Was empiric therapy given within 8 hours of arrival at hospital?

_____ Yes
_____ No, variance justified, please comment
_____ No, variance unjustified

Comment: ____

Indicator: Was empiric therapy given within 8 hours of diagnosis of CAP?

_____ Yes
_____ No, variance justified, please comment
_____ No, variance unjustified

Comment: ____

CANDIDATE FOR SWITCH THERAPY

Criteria for Switch Therapy (Put ✔ in box when Yes)

	Day 0	Day 1	Day 2	Day 3	Day 4	Day 5	Day 6	Day 7	Day >7 or NK
1. Cough & SOB improving									
2. Afebrile for ≥ 8 hours (<37.8°C, <100°F)									
3. WBC improving (↓ > 10%)									
4. Intake and absorption adequate									

To use the table, begin at day 0, which is the day of admission (or, in rare cases, the day of diagnosis) that begins at the time of admission (or time of CAP diagnosis) and ends at midnight that evening. On day 0, leave blank for present and ✔ for absent.

Day 1 begins at 00:01 and ends at midnight. On days 1 through 7, answer Cough and SOB improving and WBC count improving in comparison to the day before. ✔ the box if patient is improving or is back to baseline (before this illness).

The patient has met criteria for switch therapy when all four cells on a particular day have ✔ in them. If the patient does not meet all four criteria by day 7, the patient is not a candidate for switch therapy.

If patient dies before reaching a criterion, check NK box.

Comment: ____

Antibiotics received after switch to oral therapy

Antimicrobial	Dose/Frequency	Start Date	Stop Date

Indicator: Was switch therapy performed?

_____ Yes
_____ No, variance justified, no oral antibiotic available
_____ No, variance justified, please comment
_____ No, variance unjustified

Comment: ____________________

Indicator: Was the oral antibiotic in compliance with guidelines?

_____ Yes
_____ No, variance justified, please comment
_____ No, variance unjustified

Comment: ____________________

Once the patient was switched to oral antibiotics, was it necessary to switch back to intravenous antibiotics?

_____ No
_____ Yes, due to relapse of CAP
_____ Yes, due to other reasons, e.g. other infection, patient being NPO, etc.

Comment: ____________________

CANDIDATE FOR HOSPITAL DISCHARGE

Criteria for Hospital Discharge (Put ✔ in box when Yes)

	Day 0	Day 1	Day 2	Day 3	Day 4	Day 5	Day 6	Day 7	Day >7 or NK
1. Candidate for oral therapy									
2. Diagnostic work-up complete									
3. Comorbidity treated									
4. Social needs met									

1. (Candidate for oral therapy) should be left blank for no until all four criteria for switch therapy are met (see table, in section "Candidate for Switch Therapy"). When the patient meets criteria for switch therapy, enter ✔ for yes. Leave blank for no or ✔ for yes for the remaining categories.

When all four spaces in the column of a day are filled with ✔, the patient has met criteria for hospital discharge.

If patient dies before reaching a criterion, check NK box.

Comment: ____________________

Indicator: Was the length of hospital stay appropriate? (Discharged <24 hours after patient has met criteria for hospital discharge)

_____ Yes, length of stay was due to treatment of community-acquired pneumonia (discharged less than 24 hours after criteria for switch to oral therapy was met)
_____ Yes, length of stay was due to treatment of comorbidity
_____ Yes, length of stay was due to diagnostic work-up
_____ Yes, length of stay was due to social needs
_____ Yes, length of stay was due to other reason
_____ No, variance unjustified, switch to oral therapy not performed
_____ No, variance unjustified, switch to oral was delayed
_____ No, variance unjustified, observation on oral therapy
_____ No, variance unjustified, delayed diagnostic testing
_____ No, variance unjustified, delayed consultation
_____ No, variance unjustified, delayed social support
_____ No, variance unjustified

Comment: ____________________

CLINICAL OUTCOME

Indicator: Was early clinical outcome evaluated?

_____ Yes
_____ No, variance justified, please comment
_____ No, variance unjustified

Comment: ____________________

Indicator: Was final clinical outcome evaluated?

_____ Yes
_____ No, variance justified, patient did not return to clinic
_____ No, variance justified, unable to contact patient by phone
_____ No, variance justified, please comment
_____ No, variance unjustified

Comment: ____________________

What was the clinical outcome at final follow-up?

_____ Cured
_____ Improved
_____ Failure (check one):
    _____ Relapse of CAP
    _____ Death due to CAP
    _____ Death unrelated to CAP
    _____ Death unknown cause
    _____ Other, please comment
_____ Unknown

Comment: ____________________

PATIENT SATISFACTION WITH CARE

Indicator: Was satisfaction with care evaluated?

_____ Yes
_____ No, variance justified, patient did not return to clinic
_____ No, variance justified, unable to contact patient by phone
_____ No, variance justified, please comment
_____ No, variance unjustified

Comment: ____

Indicator: Did patient believe he/she was sent home too soon?

_____ Yes
_____ No

Comment: ____

Indicator: Did patient believe he/she received adequate follow-up care?

_____ Yes
_____ No

Comment: ____

Indicator: Was patient satisfied with the care he/she received?

_____ Yes
_____ No

Comment: ____

PREVENTION OF COMMUNITY-ACQUIRED PNEUMONIA

Indicator: Was the patient given pneumococcal vaccination?

_____ Yes
_____ No, variance justified, patient was screened but did not qualify
_____ No, variance justified, please comment
_____ No, variance unjustified

Comment: ____

Indicator: Was the patient given influenza vaccination?

_____ Yes
_____ No, variance justified, patient was screened but did not qualify
_____ No, variance justified, please comment
_____ No, variance unjustified

Comment: ____

Indicator: In patients who smoke, was smoking cessation offered?

_____ Yes
_____ Not applicable, patient does not smoke
_____ No, variance justified, please comment
_____ No, variance unjustified

Comment: ____

Subject Index

Note: Page numbers followed by f indicate figures; page numbers followed by t indicate tables.

Acid-fast bacilli, smears/cultures for, in TB workup, 18, 19, 56
Admission decision, and hospitalization for CAP, 15. *See also* Hospitalization.
Alveolar space, entry of microorganisms into, 8, 9f. *See also* Pneumonia.
Antimicrobial-resistant organisms, therapy for CAP in presence of, 25, 26t
Antimicrobial therapy, for community-acquired pneumonia, 24–29
  practice of, evaluation of, 28
    reasons for variance from, 29, 58, 60
  problems with, 47–48
  response to, 30, 45
    recovery phase in, 30
      and clinical improvement, 30, 45
    temporal variations in, 44f
  selection of, when patient is in general ward, 25, 25t, 26t
    when patient is in ICU, 26, 27t
  switch from intravenous to oral agents in, 30–34, 31f, 32f, 33f
    criteria for, 32, 59
    practice of, evaluation of, 33–34
      variance from, 34, 60
Antipseudomonal therapy, for community-acquired pneumonia, 26, 27t
Anti-smoking programs, in prevention of CAP, 49–50

Bacilli, acid-fast, on smears/cultures used in TB workup, 18, 19, 56
Blood culture results, in workup of patient with CAP, 23, 57

CAP. *See* Community-acquired pneumonia (CAP).
Chest radiography, in diagnosis of CAP, 10
Cigarette smoking, cessation of, in prevention of CAP, 49–50
Clinical course, of CAP, in hospitalized patient, 45f, 45–48
  deterioration during, 45f, 46–48
    despite antimicrobial therapy, 47–48
  improvement during, 30, 31f, 45, 45f, 46
  risk factors complicating, 14t, 54–55
Clinical outcome, of hospitalization for CAP, 43–48. *See also* Clinical course, of CAP.
  evaluation of, 48
    variance from practice of, 48, 61
Community-acquired pneumonia (CAP), 1–63. *See also* Pneumonia.
  control of, areas of management in, 3f
  indices of. *See* Quality indicator(s).
  national guidelines on, 1
    local implementation of, 1, 7f
  diagnosis of, 10
  laboratory findings in, 22
  variance from practice of, 11
    reasons for, 52
  etiology of, 21, 22t
  hospitalization for, 13–16
  admission decision and, 15
  antimicrobial therapy during. *See* Antimicrobial therapy.
  clinical outcome of, 43–48. *See also* Clinical course, of CAP.
    evaluation of, 48
      variance from practice of, 48, 61
  deterioration during, 45f, 46–48
    despite antimicrobial therapy, 47–48
  discharge concluding. *See* Discharge, of patient hospitalized for CAP.
  duration of, 35–39
    as quality indicator, 39, 61
  improvement during, 30, 31f, 45, 45f, 46
  intensive care in, antimicrobial therapy during, 26, 27t
  microbiologic workup during, 22
    variance from practice of, reasons for, 23, 57
  practice of, 6
    variance from, reasons for, 16, 54, 55

resource utilization during, 36–39, 37f, 38f
respiratory isolation in, 18–19
variance from practice of, reasons for, 19, 56
team approach to, 2
management of. *See* Community-acquired pneumonia, control of.
patient education regarding, 6, 40
practice of, evaluation of, 41
variance from, reasons for, 42, 58
patient satisfaction with care for, evaluation of, 41
results of, considered as quality indicators, 41, 62
prevention of, 49–50
practice of, evaluation of, 50
variance from, 50, 62–63
recovery from, after initiation of antimicrobial therapy, 30
risk factors complicating course of, 14t, 54–55
severity of, indices of, 14, 15t, 53–54
tuberculosis presenting as, 17–18
respiratory isolation for, 18–19
variance from practice of, reasons for, 19, 56
vs. nosocomial pneumonia, 11
Culture results, in TB workup, 18, 19, 56
in workup of patient with CAP, 23, 57

Discharge, of patient hospitalized for CAP, 35–39. *See also* Hospitalization.
criteria for, 36, 60
practice of, evaluation of, 39
variance from, 39

Education, of patient with CAP, 6, 40
practice of, evaluation of, 41
variance from, reasons for, 42, 58
Empiric antimicrobial therapy, for CAP. *See* Antimicrobial therapy.

Flu (influenza), immunization against, in prevention of CAP, 49, 50

General ward patient. *See also* Hospitalization.
CAP in, antimicrobial therapy for, 25, 25t, 26t
Gram stain, in workup of patient with CAP, 22, 57

Hospital-acquired pneumonia, vs. community-acquired pneumonia, 11

Hospitalization, for CAP, 13–16
admission decision and, 15
antimicrobial therapy during. *See* Antimicrobial therapy.
clinical outcome of, 43–48. *See also* Clinical course, of CAP.
evaluation of, 48
variance from practice of, 48, 61
deterioration during, 45f, 46–48
despite antimicrobial therapy, 47–48
discharge concluding. *See* Discharge, of patient hospitalized for CAP.
duration of, 35–39
as quality indicator, 39, 61
improvement during, 30, 31f, 45, 45f, 46
intensive care in, antimicrobial therapy during, 26, 27t
microbiologic workup during, 22
variance from practice of, reasons for, 23, 57
practice of, 6
variance from, reasons for, 16, 54, 55
resource utilization during, 36–39, 37f, 38f
respiratory isolation in, 18–19
variance from practice of, reasons for, 19, 56
team approach to, 2

Immunization, against influenza, in prevention of CAP, 49, 50
against pneumococcal pneumonia, 49, 50
Inflammatory response, in pneumonia, 8, 10, 10f, 47f
Influenza, immunization against, in prevention of CAP, 49, 50
Intensive care. *See also* Hospitalization.
for CAP, antimicrobial therapy during, 26, 27t
Intravenous antimicrobial therapy, for CAP, switch to oral agents from, 30–34, 31f, 32f, 33f
criteria for, 32, 59
practice of, evaluation of, 33–34
variance from, 34, 60
Isolation. *See also* Hospitalization.
for tuberculosis presenting as CAP, 18–19
variance from practice of, reasons for, 19, 56

Laboratory workup, during hospitalization for CAP, 22
variance from practice of, reasons for, 23, 57
Local implementation, of national guidelines on management of CAP, 1, 7f

Lung(s), infection of. *See* Pneumonia; Community-acquired pneumonia (CAP).

Microbiologic workup, during hospitalization for CAP, 22
  variance from practice of, reasons for, 23, 57
Mycobacterium tuberculosis infection, pneumonia due to, 17–18
  respiratory isolation for, 18–19
    variance from practice of, reasons for, 19, 56
  risk factors associated with, 18t

National guidelines, on management of CAP, 1
  local implementation of, 1, 7f
Nosocomial pneumonia, vs. community-acquired pneumonia, 11

Oral antimicrobial therapy, for CAP, switch from intravenous agents to, 30–34, 31f, 32f, 33f
    criteria for, 32, 59
    practice of, evaluation of, 33–34
      variance from, 34, 60
Outcome, clinical, of hospitalization for CAP, 43–48. *See also* Clinical course, of CAP.
    evaluation of, 48
      variance from practice of, 48, 61

Patient education, regarding CAP, 6, 40
  practice of, evaluation of, 41
    variance from, reasons for, 42, 58
Patient satisfaction, with care for CAP, evaluation of, 41
    results of, considered as quality indicators, 41, 62
Pneumococcal pneumonia, immunization against, 49, 50
Pneumonia, community-acquired. *See* Community-acquired pneumonia (CAP).
  etiology/pathogenesis of, 8, 9f, 21, 22t
  hospital-acquired, vs. community-acquired pneumonia, 11
  inflammatory response in, 8, 10, 10f, 47f
  influenza and, 49
  manifestations of, 10, 10f
  nosocomial, vs. community-acquired pneumonia, 11
  pathogenesis/etiology of, 8, 9f, 21, 22t
  pneumococcal, immunization against, 49, 50
  Pseudomonas aeruginosa infection and, antimicrobials effective against, 26, 27t
Pneumonia syndrome, 8, 10. *See also* Pneumonia.
  manifestations of, 10, 10f
Pseudomonas aeruginosa infection, antimicrobials effective against, 26, 27t
Pulmonary infection. *See* Pneumonia; Community-acquired pneumonia (CAP).

Quality indicator(s), of control of CAP, 4–5
  diagnosis-related, 11, 52
    workup results as, 22–23, 57
  outcome-oriented, 48, 61
  patient-based, 41–42, 58, 62
  prevention-related, 50, 62–63
  treatment-related, 19, 28, 34, 37, 56, 58, 59, 60
    hospitalization criteria and, 54, 55

Radiography, of chest, in diagnosis of CAP, 10
Recovery, from CAP, after initiation of antimicrobial therapy, 30
Resistance, antimicrobial, therapy for CAP in presence of, 25, 26t
Resource utilization, during hospitalization for CAP, 36–39, 37f, 38f
Respiratory isolation. *See also* Hospitalization.
  for tuberculosis presenting as CAP, 18–19
  variance from practice of, reasons for, 19, 56

Smears, for acid-fast bacilli, in TB workup, 18, 19, 56
Smoking cessation, in prevention of CAP, 49–50
Sputum sample studies, results of, in TB workup, 18
  in workup of patient with CAP, 22, 57
Streptococcus pneumoniae infection, immunization against, 49, 50
Switch therapy, in antimicrobial management of CAP, 30–34, 31f, 32f, 33f
  criteria for, 32, 59
  practice of, evaluation of, 33–34
    variance from, 34, 60

TB. *See* Tuberculosis.
Team approach, to hospitalization for CAP, 2
Tobacco use, cessation of, in prevention of CAP, 49–50

Tuberculosis, pneumonia due to, 17–18
respiratory isolation for, 18–19
variance from practice of, reasons for, 19, 56
risk factors associated with, 18t

Vaccination, against influenza, in prevention of CAP, 49, 50
against pneumococcal pneumonia, 49, 50

Variance from practice, in control of CAP. *See* Quality indicator(s).

Ward patient. *See also* Hospitalization.
CAP in, antimicrobial therapy for, 25, 25t, 26t

X-ray study, of chest, in diagnosis of CAP, 10